Doctor Help Me Slim Down!

Doctor Help Me Slim Down!

Firm up and get rid of cellulite!

Dr. Maria Makarovic

Writer's Showcase
New York Lincoln Shanghai

Doctor Help Me Slim Down!
Firm up and get rid of cellulite!

Writer's Showcase
an imprint of iUniverse, Inc.

For information address:
iUniverse
2021 Pine Lake Road, Suite 100
Lincoln, NE 68512
www.iuniverse.com

ISBN: 0-595-24564-1

Printed in the United States of America

Contents

Introduction

Never like in the last few years has the battle against cellulite and excess weight appeared to have become such a major issue for millions of women of all ages. Eighty percent of the female population experiences problems linked to the presence of 'saddlebag' thighs and 'orange peel' skin after puberty. It is not just an esthetic problem but also a real disorder that involves the body tissues, blood circulation and lymphatic system. Seeking help from unqualified people without medical training can aggravate the physical problem, adding to this a significantly negative psychological factor, caused by the frustration of not being able to reach the much desired results.

On the surface of the skin cellulite appears as hollows and crater-like bulges which give the skin that typically lumpy appearance. At first, the symptoms are subtle: tingling in the legs, cold feet, show of capillaries, formation of varicose veins, culminating finally at the stage in which pain is felt when the area affected by cellulite is pinched.

Anxiousness and insecurity are often the most common psychological consequences found amongst women who suffer from this problem and cause many of them to abandon their social life and to fall into self pity.

For my patients, eliminating this fat meant finding a new life, regaining their lost enthusiasm, feeling more secure, and finally succeeding in looking at themselves as individuals rather than as "freaks of nature".

What was my role?

To lead these women to their pre-established goal—that of defeating cellulite once and for all—by advising them, comforting them, and even scolding them at the right times.

Part One

The unidentified illness
General Information

Cellulite

The scientific name for this disorder, which 'laymen' erroneously call cellulite, is *edema to-tibrosclerotic panniculopathy*. This term describes a condition that is not only ugly, but also debilitating from a physical and psychological standpoint, and defines in depth the types of damage found in the affected tissues.

Cellulite is an inflammation of the panniculus adiposus found in subcutaneous cell tissue *(hypodermis)*, composed of fat lobules *(adipocytes)* separated from another by a latticework of pre-collagen, collagen and elastic fibers.

The connective tissue between the fat cells is supplied by a dense lymphatic and capillary network whose task is to aid the exchange of nutriments between the blood and tissues.

When this vascular network is altered for any reason, there is first an accumulation of fluid in the space between the cells *(edema)*. Edema hinders local blood circulation, causing an increase in the number of connective cells, which results in the hardening of the tissue *(sclerosis)*. After this, even the inner part of the skin, the *dermis*, which connects the external epidermis with the hypodermis and which is made up of numerous nerves and sensory receptors, collagen and elastic tissue, can be affected.

If not treated, cellulite degenerates into nodular formations which are visible on the skin surface and are quite hard and painful to the touch.

Cellulite is a problem that is found predominantly in women.

The area most affected is the upper side of the thighs, corresponding to the prominence on the upper part of the femur *(trochanteric area)*. Other areas may also be affected, such as the buttocks, the inner part of the knees and inner thighs, the upper third of the leg, calves, ankles and in some cases even the breasts.

Cellulite is divided into four *stages*, or degrees, according to the degree to which it has developed:

In the FIRST STAGE there is an initial retention of liquid in the connective tissue, caused by a slowdown in the local microcirculation. In this phase the volume of the adipocytes also begins to increase. The patient feels no pain, even when the area is palpated.

In the SECOND STAGE the collagen and elastic fibers surrounding the adipocytes multiply and harden, with the resulting formation of fibrous tissue, similar to that of scars (beginning of the process leading to sclerosis). Although there is no pain, when pressing the area with a finger a very visible mark is left on the skin.

In these first two stages the skin surface appears smooth and even, has a normal color, and looks slightly swollen. Symptoms due to inadequate circulation may be present, such as tingling, heaviness and cramps in the legs, especially in the evening.

In the THIRD STAGE the connective tissue becomes even harder and begins to incorporate the fat lobules as if in a vice, preventing them from receiving adequate irroration. The tissue is considerably affected, with the formation of the first macronodules which, on the skin surface, present the characteristic 'orange peel' appearance.

In the FOURTH STAGE the fat lobules are completely encapsulated by the sclerotic tissue in fibrous cell areas, isolated from the tissue surrounding them. These nodules give rise to considerable hollows and protuberances on the skin surface, which may look like hard little beads, sometimes as big as a hazelnut, and are extremely painful. This is the most difficult form of cellulite to treat and indicates an often irreversible stage of its development. When palpated the skin feels rough (hard) and is painful; when the ankles and calves are affected, the hardening can be seen from the top of the malleolus to the calf. Most often this kind of cellulite affects the thigh area, but can also be found in other isolated areas.

In the region of the malleolus there may, at times, be a noticeable swelling due to the edema; the skin appears taught like a balloon, and when pressed it feels like one is touching a gelatinous substance and the mark left by the finger remains for a few seconds. In the calf and pre-tibia area often all four stages coexist.

Around the ankles a difference in consistency can be felt when touched lightly with a finger.

Constant pain is felt only in the third and fourth stages, and can become so acute and persistent that the patient awakes in the middle of the night. In these last two phases the elasticity of the skin diminishes to the point that it loses considerable tone (flaccidity).

Capillaries and varicose veins thus find a favorable environment in which to become evident on the skin surface.

There are, moreover, *three different kinds* of cellulite: edematous, compact, flaccid.

EDEMATOUS. This kind is frequent in the first and second stages. The skin appears puffy, lighter, and may show some spider veins in areas. It is generally accompanied by circulatory insufficiency.

COMPACT. This type may be found in all of the stages as a consequence of edematous cellulite.

FLACCID (OR FLABBY). May develop as a result of compact cellulite.

This flabbiness is visible when the patient is standing in an erect position. When the skin is pinched a considerable fold can be lifted and when this is let go there will be a noticeable drop in the tissue, It is easily found in people who are subject to a sedentary lifestyle, who went on different unbalanced lowcalorie diets or experienced drastic weight losses.

The causes of cellulite

Eighty per cent of all women are affected by cellulite. This disorder is found almost exclusively amongst the female population after adolescence. The main causes of its onset and its worsening are considered to be the following:

HEREDITARY FACTORS. It is likely that some have a genetic predisposition to cellulite if the mother or grandmother suffer from this problem. It is important to avoid other causes which may aggravate an environment already favorable to the stagnation of body fluids which then degenerates into cellulite, and to therefore avoid a sedentary lifestyle and unhealthy diet.

ESTROGEN. Female hormones foster the accumulation of fat and liquids in the buttocks, hip and thigh areas. Here, in particular, there are enzymes which enable the adipose cells to hold in a greater quantity of fat, since women, in the event of a pregnancy, will need to store up a larger energy reserve.

CONTRACEPTIVE PILL. The quantity of estrogen contained in such pills may lead to the onset of cellulite. The tissues in the thighs appear to contain greater amounts of liquid and, in the event of a greater Calorie intake, have a greater probability a localized increase of fatty tissue and cellulite.

SEDENTARY LIFESTYLE. Lack of movement hinders adequate circulation, thus causing liquids to be retained in critical points. An excessive intake of food, moreover, also causes an increase in fatty tissue. These three factors work together until over time the skin assumes that uneven appearance.

SMOKING. Too many cigarettes have a negative effect on the oxygen supply to the tissues. Consequently, it is preferable to avoid not only direct smoke, but also indirect smoke, inhaled as a result of other people smoking nearby. The harmful substances are inhaled and are introduced into the circulatory system where they prove to cause irritation to the small capillaries in particular, and in the cellulite tissue they suffer.

WINE. Provokes the dilation of the blood vessels and, consequently, causes an increase of liquid retention in the inter-cellular area. Drinking the occasional glass is not harmful, but over three glasses per day will aggravate the problem. One gram of wine contains 7 Calories, so half a liter a day corresponds to the equivalent of eating a whole plate of pasta.

TIGHT CLOTHES. It is not advisable to wear very tight-fitting jeans, underpants with too tight an elastic, too close-fitting girdles or leotards, garters or thighhigh stockings, since they hinder the circulation of the blood.

SHOES WITH HEELS OVER 4 CENTIMETERS HIGH. Heels that are too high force women to walk in an incorrect manner, with the result that the local blood circulation is impeded.

FRENETIC EXERCISE. Aerobics and running are not advisable when cellulite has reached the fourth stage. The lactic acid, produced as a result of prolonged exercise, is drained with greater difficulty because of the already affected local circulation and can even worsen the condition of the tissues.

PREGNANCY. During pregnancy, estrogen, combined with an excessive weight gain (over 25 pounds), can lead to an increase of cellulite in the thigh area. Moreover, the fetus, putting added volume on the abdominal area, increases the pressure in that area, which hinders the circulation of the veins in the lower pelvic region and, consequently, all the blood vessels stemming out from them. The blood circulation is therefore slowed down, which leads to heavy and swollen legs.

KITCHEN SALT. An excess of salt (sodium chloride) predisposes one to greater water retention, therefore it is advisable to reduce one's salt intake. Those who suffer from low blood pressure (hypotension) should eliminate it with caution.

SUPER-ALCOHOLIC DRINKS. An excessive amount of super-alcoholic drinks, in addition to causing a surplus Calorie intake, does not supply any essential nutritional substances such as vitamins and minerals, and places an incredibly heavy burden on the liver, thus making digestion more difficult.

CONSTIPATION. When suffering from constipation, the toxins produced by the by-products of digestion remain in the intestines longer. It is important therefore to add foods to one's diet that contain fiber, in order to increase the peristalsis of the intestines and thereby quicken evacuation.

CONSTIPATION

We usually speak of constipation when the intestine does not empty itself for three to four days, or when the frequency of evacuation is less than twice a week. Naturally, this statement is based on biological statistics, but every individual must be assessed according to subjective criteria, because physical problems may occur within a shorter time too, for example after one day. The symptoms range from stomach pain to bloatedness, which may even lead to the outbreak of hemorrhoids due to increased abdominal pressure and the effort required to have a bowel movement.

When constipation occurs, many resort to an inordinate use of laxatives. These irritate the inner lining of the intestines and thus stimulate in an unnatural manner. When using the plant-based kinds, one must check whether they contain Senna or Aloe, because these can lead to tolerance and then greater doses will be required for the same effect. To solve the problem, it is advisable to walk for at least one hour per day, drink two liters of water throughout the day and eat fiber-rich foods, such as fruit and vegetables, bran and other roughage. The latter type of fiber increases the volume and soften the feces.

Aggravating factors

In addition to the causes already mentioned, there are other factors that influence the formation of cellulite and aggravate some conditions related to cellulite, and which are closely linked to the female hormonal cycle.

One of the moments when the problems linked to cellulite seem to worsen is during the so-called PREMENSTRUAL SYNDROME. This consists in a series of somatic disorders and mood swings, recurring during the progesterone phase of the menstrual cycle. The insatiable urge for carbohydrates or fatty foods is one aspect that is found amongst a minority of women.

The explanation for this is not entirely clear; it seems that the metabolism of the hormone called *serotonine is* involved, and perhaps the *melatonine* about which there is so much talk recently.

Often women prone to this syndrome experience what is known as seasonal pattern bulimia.; a slight increase of appetite is, therefore, to be considered normal, whereas a sensation of uncontrollable "hunger" is to be seen as a problem requiring medical or psychological assistance.

These crises cause a weight gain if there is a food intake, but sometimes when the menstrual cycle is nearing, a woman may weigh as much as 3 pounds more because of the water retention induced by the action of the hormones in the body's center of gravity (thighs and hips).

During the MENSTRUAL CYCLE certain psycho-physical conditions recurring with a certain frequency in women who have a problem with cellulite and excess weight may also become more evident, such as fatigue and depression. These are further accentuated in women who have a lack of iron. Women who still have their menstrual cycle can easily compensate for this deficiency: during their period women lose about 13 mg of iron daily, whereas the other days they lose about 5 mg, just like men. A blood test will determine the amount of iron there is in the blood (siderimia). An iron deficiency gives rise to muscular and psychological fatigue, in addition to causing hair and nails to become fragile.

IRON: AN ESSENTIAL MINERAL

A scientific study was carried out on the link between iron intake and scholastic performance. In fact, the results were quite significant: an iron deficiency causes students to become listless and makes them more prone to infections.

Another moment when excess weight is lurking is MENOPAUSE, the natural process by which the ovaries gradually lose their ability to produce estrogen, the female sex hormones. This usually occurs between ages 45 and 50, when women cease to have their menstrual cycle. During this phase, many women gain weight because, as their metabolism slows down, the adipose tissue tends to increase, and is compounded by a lack of physical activity.

In order to ease the discomfort that accompanies menopause, hormone therapy has some considerable advantages:

—it reduces heat flashes

—reduces atrophy of the vagina

—has a beneficial effect on the skin

—prevents osteoporosis and heart attack

—improves memory and sexual intercourse.

Taking hormone supplements may cause some water retention, but the discomfort may be attenuated or even eliminated by eating plenty of fruits and vegetables.

Weight gain may be kept under control with a balanced diet and adequate physical exercise. A diet lacking in *protein* from milk, meat, fish and eggs will lead to an insufficient production of muscle mass with the resulting tendency towards plumpness.

For those who prefer to follow a vegetarian diet, it is advisable that they seek advice from a specialist, so as not to run the risk of eating foods with the right amount of amino acids and vitamin B12.

A warm-up suit and a pair of jogging shoes will help in maintaining good muscle tone.

The remedies

There are a variety of ways to prevent the onset of cellulite and to help in eliminating this problem. In addition to *exercising* and *dieting*, there are a number of medical therapies that are particularly suitable for women who suffer from cellulite in its less advanced stages, including *mesotherapy, ultrasound therapy, laser therapy, magnetic therapy,* and *electro-toning therapy, to* be utilized under the close observation of a specialist, which, especially if several of these methods are employed in combination, guarantee excellent results already after the first few sessions.

EXCESS WEIGHT AND OBESITY

The term *excess weight* indicates an increase in body weight ranging between 10 and 20% over the ideal weight of an individual. When the weight gain exceeds 20% of the ideal weight, we begin speaking of *obesity*

Why do people gain weight? Living in an affluent society leads to greater possibilities for eating and therefore to an excess of calories to the detriment of food quality. For most people who struggle with weight problems, the cause of their weight gain is a calorie intake that exceeds the amount their body consumes.

The battle against excess weight becomes almost a necessity in that, in the case of obesity, it increases the predisposition to be at risk for medical complications such as hypertension, glucose intolerance, diabetes, cardiovascular disease, hypertriglyceridemia, hyperuricemia and certain types of cancer (colon, breast).

In evaluating obesity it is essential not only to quantify the excess weight, but also to determine where the adipose tissue is distributed throughout the body. In particular, it was found that fat distribution in the visceral, or inner abdominal, area is greatly associated with the prevalence of diabetes, high blood pressure and hypercholesterolemia (all risk factors for vascular disease), particularly evident in young adults. Moreover, excess weight is associated with an increased mortality rate in both men and women.

Treatment by means of a diet may be sufficient to prevent and normalize these parameters, which are otherwise modified only with the prescription of certain drugs.

Defining obesity

Obesity is often, generically, considered an excess of weight or body fat. Actually, no single definition has yet been found, and as such many different reference levels exist. Obesity may therefore be defined as:

A CERTAIN DEGREE OF EXCESS WEIGHT. Obesity may be considered an excess of

caption pg. 1 8

OBESITY AND BLOOD PRESSURE

An obese person has larger adipose cells, which make it more difficult for the blood to circulate. The blood volume in circulation, as a consequence, increases, and this may raise both the maximum and the minimum pressure in that there is a greater resistance of the venous blood.

weight above an optimal level, in accordance with height/weight tables or the Body Mass Index (BMI).

A HIGH DEGREE OF EXCESS WEIGHT. Some researchers use a range for ideal weight, excess weight and obesity. In this definition, excess weight generally means 110-119% above one's ideal weight, and obesity is considered as 120% or more. Obesity may also refer to a BMI equal to 30 or to higher figures, whereas excess weight may even indicate a lower BMI. This definition, however, is less commonly used.

A HIGH DEGREE OF ADIPOSE TISSUE OR BODY FAT. Obesity is often defined as a surplus of body fat, in some cases regardless of weight.

A HIGH DEGREE OF HEALTH RISK. An ideal definition, according to some experts, would consist in determining the point beyond which an excess of fat or weight would put the health of the individual at risk.

Actually, this definition creates some problems:

—the reference point is not known, and even if it were, it would probably differ according to a number of variables, such as genetic factors, fat distribution, eating habits, lifestyle and physical activity;

—obesity is not exclusively a health issue, it also involves political and social factors.

The term 'obesity' comes from Latin and is correlated to the meaning of the verb 'to eat' (edere), but this etymological view does not take into consideration the complexity of the causes of this problem and is as such a rather unsatisfactory term.

Often, at the social level moreover, there is an improper use of the word 'obesity', which lends it an overly broad significance, thereby penalizing patients affected by general problems of excess weight. It is better for the term 'obese' to be used as an adjective, and not as a reference to a particular group of people (the 'obese group' and the 'non-obese group'), and for the expression 'serious obesity' to indicate only values referring to a BMI above 40.

DAMAGE FROM VISCERAL OBESITY

With visceral obesity a greater amount of free fatty acids (FFA) is sent straight to the liver. These are produced by the breakdown of triglycerides and, when processed by the liver, cause a reduction in the clearance of insulin, producing, as a result, an increase (hyperinsulinemia) of insulin in the blood. This causes the amount of LDL (the so-called 'bad' cholesterol) to increase, and reduces the amount of HDL ('good' cholesterol), which may subsequently give rise to an intolerance to insulin and a propensity for diabetes. Hyperinsufnemia causes hypertension, because it causes a rise in the exchangeable body sodium, due to an altered secretion of and resistance to natruretic atrial peptide (hormone secreted in the atrial lining of the heart). This explains why obese individuals, even if they reduce their kitchen salt intake, do not show major improvements in their blood pressure, but need to lose weight.

How to calculate one's ideal weight and measure obesity

The simplest way to determine your ideal weight is to consult the table below

HEIGHT/WEIGHT TABLE

STATURE meters	WOMEN	MEN	WEIGHT kg IMC
	Serious obesity	Serious obesity	
	Medium obesity	Medium obesity	
	Excess weight	Excess weight	
	NORMAL	NORMAL	
	Underweight	Underweight	

With a ruler you connect the two points corresponding to your own weight and height, which are found respectively in the column on the right (weight) and the column on the left (height) of the table. The meeting point between the middle line and the line traced by the ruler will show the range in which your weight falls.

caption pg. 20

WOMEN Age (years)	Height (cm)	Weight (kg)
17	163	56
18-29	162	55
30-59	161	54
> 60	159	52

MEN

Age (years)	Height (cm)	Weight (kg)
17	174	67
18-29	175	67
30-59	171	65
> 60	169	63

By using the ratio between weight and height, we also calculate the BMI (body mass index), which is widely used in research all over the world. Its greatest advantages are that it is objective, repeatable and can be used to quantify and compare different data.

For a person to be considered of normal weight, the BMI values must fall within the following parameters, which differ for men and women:

$BMI = Kg/m^2$

	Man	woman
Normal range	19.5-24.5	18.5-23
Figures above this range indicate excess weight or obesity		
Excess weight	24.5-30	23-28
Medium obesity	30-40	28-40
Serious obesity	≥ 40	

It should not be forgotten that obesity is measured in various ways depending on whether one refers to medicine, to studies on this phenomenon and the causes of epidemics or to research.

The standard method of calculation is the height/weight ratio method. These measurements are then taken to calculate optimal weight utilizing the height/weight table, or the BMI range by means of the simple weight/height (kg/sq. m.) calculation.

The height/weight tables are easier to understand by the general public and therefore by patients.

The new US standard for height/weight tables is found in the *Acceptable Weights for Men and Women, from 1991 Dietary Guidelines for Americans (USDA)*. Unfortunately, there is a lack of such clear and widely accepted guidelines for Italians.

This USDA table offers a weight range with reference to the past, which is why men and women are placed in the same category. This allows for a higher weight range for persons age 35 or above.

The Metropolitan Life Insurance Company has produced, since 1942, reference tables for ideal weight, published in journals in 1983. Numerous experts today prefer to use tables published in 1959.

Another method of determining excess body fat is to calculate the patient's ANTHROMETRIC MEASUREMENTS by measuring the circumferences of specific body parts of the patient. These measurements are commonly used to determine the distribution of fat in the body and the risk of fat in the abdominal area.

The waist/hip ratio corresponds to the measurement of the circumference of the waist over the widest circumference of the hips. The distribution of fat according to this ratio (Vague, Bionthorpe and others) is considered an indicator of pathologies linked to obesity. A low risk is established around a level of 0.95 or lower for men and 0.8 or lower for women, in accordance with *USDA 1999 Dietary Guidelines for Americans*. The risk is considered greater when these levels are exceeded.

As you will notice, this method of measurement does not indicate the actual percentage of body fat or its distribution in the abdominal region. Thus, the issue of a pathological risk remains open in that the risk is closely correlated, not so much to an excess of weight or to a constitutional biotype, as to the fat mass and to the distribution of this fat in the abdominal region. It is therefore necessary to determine the body composition in order to obtain a better assess any pathological risk.

Where anthropometric measurements are taken

The circumference of the waist must be measured at the half-way point between the last rib and the uppermost part of the hipbone (iliac crest).

The circumference of the *hips is* measured on the boney prominence at the upper part of the femur (great trochanters).

The circumference of the *thighs is* measured at the height of the buttocks.

wrist
arm
waist
hips
thigh
knee (above rotula) knee (below rotula)
calf
ankle

Types of obesity

Obesity is classified according to its causes or origin (essential or endocrine) and to the distribution of fat throughout the body (android or gynecoid).

Essential or endocrine obesity

As far as the causes of its appearance are concerned, obesity can be labeled as either essential or endocrine (secondary).

ESSENTIAL OBESITY (hyperplastic or hypertrophic) is the frequent kind. In this case there is an increase in the volume and number of adipocytes, generally due to a difference between the quantity of calories consumed and the daily energy requirements of a given individual. This often begins during infancy, but may also arise in adults, as a consequence of a psychological condition.

ENDOCRINE OBESITY occurs as a result of illnesses involving alterations at a glandular level *(endocrinopathy)*, such as the Cushing syndrome, hypothyroidism, diabetes, ovarian polycystosis, hypothalamo—hypophysa injury, or from taking particular drugs (contraceptives, cortizones).

Android or gynoid obesity

In terms of the distribution of fat tissue, we speak of

ABDOMINAL OR CENTRAL OR ANDROID OBESITY when the waist/hips ratio (WHIR) is > 0.85;

GLUTEO-FEMORAL OR PERIPHERAL OR GYNECOID OBESITY when the waist/hips ratio (WHIR) is < 0.78.

The adipose tissue (body fat) may be located mainly in abdominal region—and in this case we speak of *android obesity*, because it is found more frequently in men, whose sex hormones, androgens, have different functions compared to female estrogen—or in the glutei-femoral region (in the hips and thigh area)—and thus we speak of *gynecoid obesity*, because it is more frequent among women. In the latter case, when weight is lost, it is more difficult to lose centimeters around the hips, buttocks and thighs, and cellulite can begin to be a visible problem. Research has demonstrated that in the thigh region there is a higher number of 'switches' (Alpha 2 receptors) that enable adipose cells to absorb fatty acids more easily. Estrogen, during the premenstrual period, causes even more liquid to be retained in the area of the hips, and the problem is further accentuated if the contraceptive pill is taken.

In abdominal fat deposits, a distinction is made between the subcutaneous component and the visceral component. With the exact same waistline, men usually accumulate fat in the intravisceral region—a factor increasingly correlated to the likelihood of a heart attack—while women tend to have a greater quantity of subcutaneous adipose tissue. It is possible for this tissue to undergo an alteration in the process of its fat metabolism *(lipodystrophy)*.

The remedies

In the abdominal region, where adipose tissue can easily evolve into cellulite, the most effective therapy among women is *mesotherapy,* whenever dieting alone is not sufficient to show noticeable results and improved looks. This method involves the use of pharmaceutical products which dissolve fat *(lipolytic solutions)*. In men, subcutaneous fat is less present, so after losing some weight each case must be dealt with more individual attention.

Anti-appetite medication

These are pharmaceutical products that lessen the sensation of hunger, by stimulating the sensory center of satiety or inhibiting the hunger sensors. They are often utilized in combination with psychological therapy.

It is advisable to prescribe them to patients with a BMI > 30, in cases where low-calorie diets have produced no weight loss. The use of such drugs is opted for when the pounds to lose are more difficult, in that they are not liquid but rather only pure fat.

FLUOXETINE. Acts as an anti-depressant. It may be administered by a psychiatrist or by a specialist to counteract an obsessive sense of hunger. *Contraindications:* hypersensitivity to its components; use of other antidepressants **(IMAO); kidney** or liver disease, diabetes, pregnancy, nursing mothers.

FENDIMETRAZINE An amphetamine used in therapies to complement a diet. *Contraindication:* hypersensitivity to its components, arterial pulmonary hypertension, arterial hypertension, card io-cerebrovascular disease,

Caption pg. 25

Mesotherapy
pg. 200—Of

arteriosclerosis, hyperthyroidism, glaucoma, nervousness, pregnancy, nursing mothers. Do not administer to children under age 12.

DEXFENFLUORAMINE:. This is a serotoninergic k_ dug that acts en the medial nuclei of the hypothalamo, also called the 'hunger center'. It acts in particular to reduce the intake of sugar-rich foods. It does not have the effect of a psychostimulant.

Contraindications: known hypersensitivity to this drug, pregnancy, breastfeeding, glaucoma, in combination with ether antidepressants (IMAO), arterial pulmonary hypertension, cerebro-vascular disease, psychiatric illness, nervous anorexia, liver or kidney failure.

Natural substances that assist the metabolism of fat

In addition to anti-appetite drugs, there are certain natural substances that can be introduced in a low-calorie diet to help the body metabolize fats and facilitate digestion.

OMEGA 3 POLYUNSATURATED FATTY ACIDS. These are very useful in the event that there is a high level of triglycerides in the bleed (hypertriglyceridemia).

CHITOSAN. This is an aminopolysaccaride derived from chitin, a natural substance found in the shells of marine shellfish. It causes the fat and cholesterol ingested along with food to be channeled to the intestine, so a part these substances cannot be absorbed and are eliminated.

It is net recommended for these who are allergic to shellfish, for these with gastrointestinal illnesses or who take certain drugs, such as the pill, which cannot be absorbed properly.

CHROME PICOLINATE. Based en a scientific study carried out by the Clinic of San Antonio, Texas, it was found that in patients to whom this substance was administered there was a less of fatty tissue and an increase of muscle tissue. Chrome picolinate is the active ingredient of chrome. It festers the synthesis of muscle volume and diminishes the urge to eat sweets. Its action causes the body tissues to be sensitized to insulin. In fat people the increase of the adipocytes (fat cells) reduces the sensitivity to this hormone.

DEXTRAN. Any of a number of polysaccarides that reduce the absorption of fat in the intestines.

PANCREATIN. A mixture of enzymes extracted from the pancreatic juice, containing principally amylase, trypsin, and lipase, which help in the digestion of starches, proteins and lipids.

Nutrients and diet

The human body requires a regular supply of energy. This is provided by the foods that are eaten and which contain substances that serves to form, develop and renew body tissues (bones, muscle, nerves, etc.). These substances are defined as *nutrients* and the principal ones are:

> PROTEINS OR PROTIDES1 gr. supplies 4 Calories
> SUGARS OR GLUCIDES OR CARBO-HYDRATES 1 gr. supplies 4 Calories

FATS OR LIPIDS 1 gr. supplies 9 Calories
VITAMINS 0 Calories
MINERALS 0 Calories
WATER 0 Calories
ETHYL ALCOHOL 1 gr. supplies 7 Calories

Protein

Protein plays an important role in the growth and repair of tissue (plastic function), for the elasticity of skin and proper muscle trophism. They are formed by a series of combinations of *amino acids*, which contain the elements of carbon, hydrogen, oxygen, nitrogen and sometimes even sulfur.

There are two groups of amino acids, the *essential* and the *non-essential*. The former are called essential, because our organism is not able to produce them and they must therefore be supplied by ingesting foods. The second kind are synthesized by our body from a series of other components.

In order for these to be utilized properly from a biochemical standpoint, it is absolutely necessary that the amino acids be combined with the right amount of glucides *(simple sugars,* such as table sugar, honey, and *complex sugars,* such

ESSENTIAL AMINO ACIDS

Arginine	Indispensable for optimal growth, since it stimulates the growth hormone, increases muscle volume reducing the fat level, stimulates the immune system and helps the cicatrization process.
Histidine threonine ptophan	
Isoleucine, Leucine and Valine	Important in the production of both red and white blood cells.
Methionine Phenylalanine	An important element of collagen, the protein that is the chief constituent of the fibrils of connective tissue, such as skin. It is not found in vegetarian diets. Tryptophan is utilized by the brain to produce serotonin, which has an effect against stress, hunger, anxiousness and depression. In some cases it may be useful in reducing headaches.
	Metabolized principally in the muscles and not in the liver as are the others. The body requires balanced proportions of these.
	Helps to fight against hair loss. Has a beneficial effect on a person's mood

NON-ESSENTIAL AMINO ACIDS

Aspartic acid Glutamic acid	is implemented in the transformation of RNA and DNA.
	is involved in the brain's metabolic mechanisms, fights against stress, fatigue poor concentration. It also has the function of transporting potassium. Necessary for the growth of hair.
Cistine and Cisteine Tyrosine	The precursor of a hormone called noradrenaline, which is effective in educing appetite.

as pasta, bread, rice and potatoes); this way the body can store the protein and thus maintain good muscle tone or increase the muscle volume.

Sugars

The energy supplied by glucides is metabolized rapidly by all the tissue (the brain requires 100 gr. of glucose per day). In order for these glucides to be utilized by the body, they must be transformed into glucose, sugar in its most simple state, which is involved in the biochemical processes of living cells.

Nearly all sugars are composed of glucose molecules or of similar molecules such as fructose (fruit) and galactose (milk). These molecules, when combined, form chains, and the longer and more complex they are, the longer the process will be a breaking them down into glucose in order to be absorbed by the body. Depending on the length of the molecular chain, therefore, we have sugar that are absorbed very rapidly, rapidly or slowly.

The very rapidly absorbed sugars (5 minutes) include simple sugars (monosaccharides), composed of a single molecule of 6 carbon atoms.

NAME	FOODS THAT CONTAIN
THEM Glucose Grapes-Honey Fructose	Fruit-Honey
Galactose	Milk

The rapidly absorbed sugars (10 minutes) include sugars that are composed of two molecules of simple sugars *(disaccharides)*.

NAME	FOODS THAT CONTAIN
THEM Saccharose	
(glucose+fructose)	Table sugar Lactose
(glucose+galactose)	Milk and dairy products
Maltose	
(glucose+glucose)	Beer

Slowly absorbed sugars include the sugars that are composed of a chain of molecules of simple sugars (polisaccharides).

NAME	FOODS THAT CONTAIN THEM
Starch	Cereal, potatoes, pasta, bread, legumes.
Glycogen	Muscles (meat, liver).

When an excess of sugars compared to the requirements of the body is consumed, they are accumulated as a reserve in the liver and in the muscles in the form of glycogen, and in adipose tissue in the form of fat. In the event that not enough food is eaten or that the organism's calorie requirements increase, the body can then make use of these energy reserves.

Often, when dieting to lose weight, it is advisable to substitute common table sugar (saccharose) with natural or artificial sweeteners, which are very low in calories.

SWEETENERS

One serving of sweeteners, in the form of either a tablet or a bag, contain less than one Calorie. They can be taken without risk as long as the recommended daily allowance, allowance e is not exceeded.

DUCED BY LABORATORY SYNTHESIS FROM VARIOUS CHEMICAL SUBSTANCES

Artificial sweeteners have a greater sweetening capacity compared to natural ones, in particular table sugar (saccharose), even though they do not contain any Calories. They simply have to be consumed with moderation.

Saccharine

saccharine   The most widely used sweetener. It is often mixed with other sweeteners to cover its bitter aftertaste. The RDA is 2.5 mg/kg of body weight.

Cyclamate has no bitter aftertaste. The RDA is 0-4 mg/kg of body weight. D-trytophan an isomer of an essential amino acid, the toxicology is unknown. Aspartame is derived from two amino acids. Has a taste similar to that of table sugar. Should not be used by persons suffering from phenylketonuria. ptophan Aspartame tassium acesulfame Potassium acesulfame a potassium salt, with no bitter aftertaste. The RDA is 0-9 mg/kg of body weight.

PRODUCED BY LABORATORY SYNTHESIS FROM SACCHAROSE

These are natural sweeteners, and they are reconverted into glucose by the body. They all supply more or less 4 Calories per gram, even though they have a greater sweetening capacity.

Fructose (levulose or sugar from fruit Mannitol of

The kind found on the market is produced from saccharose. One serving corresponds to half a serving of saccharose, in terms of sweetness.

Found in nature in olives, figs and celery. Has a laxative effect, and for this reason is mixed with other sweeteners.

Is derived from glucose. The RDA is 30-70 g per day. May have a laxative effect.

xylitol As sweet as saccharose and appears to protect against cavities. It is tolerated by humans without a laxative effect in amounts up to 70 g per day.

Fats

Fats make up a large number of cellular structures and provide a fundamental energy reserve for the body. They make foods tastier, but also supply a large

Caption pg. 32 *KETONE BODIES*

These are compounds, such as/-hydroxybutyrric acid, acetoacetic acid and acetone, which are formed when the amount of glucose in the body is insufficient. This occurs during a fast, with a high fever and in diabetes mellitus.

amount of calories. One teaspoon of oil (10 gr.) has 90 Calories. This is why it is necessary to be very careful to not exceed the recommended amounts. When fats are used to supply energy, as occurs during a fast, they give rise to waste products *(ketone bodies)*, which in excessive quantities are eliminated in the urine (ketonuria) or in the form of bad breath (in this case, it is called acetonic breath, because it smells like rotten fruit).

Fats are also called *triglycerides* because they are composed of one molecule of glycerol and three molecules of fatty acids. These acids are also formed of a chain of carbon atoms, and the nature of the various fats is determined by the length of these chains.

The carbon atoms are connected to one another by simple (single) or double chemical bonds. If the fatty acids are composed of single bonds they are called *saturated* fats, and are generally present in animal fats. If, instead, they contain many double bonds they are called *polyunsaturated* fats, and *we* find these in vegetal fats. The greater the number of double bonds in the molecule, the easier it is for it to react to other chemical elements, particularly with the oxygen found in the air. This is why, if oil is left uncovered, it begins to oxidize and to become rancid. It then takes on a bad odor and an unpleasant taste, and for this reason should always be kept shut and away from light.

In foods, lipids may be either 'visible', as in butter, lard, margarine and oil, or 'invisible', as those found in cheese, meats, milk and eggs.

In terms of nutrition, olive oil is preferable to butter because it is rich in polyunsaturated fatty acids, which are important in preventing arteriosclerosis. Oil contains essential fatty acids, one of which in particular, linoleic acid, cannot be synthesized by our organism. This acid plays a fundamental role in the composition of cell membranes, required to maintain the cell structure intact, in addition to preventing some dermatitises and excessive dryness of the skin, and it is what prostaglandin and other hormones are synthesized from. The minimum daily requirement is 3 gr. When a person on a diet is not allowed more than two spoons of oil, then it is preferable to use corn, soybean, grapeseed or sunflower oil.

> FOR 100 gr. OF OIL=gr. OF LINOLEIC ACID
> *Olive oil=7.85 gr.*
> *Sunflower oil=49.89 gr.*
> *Corn oil=49.83 gr.*
> *Grape-seed oil=67.70 gr.*

Amongst these oils, it is better to use oil from cold-pressed olives (extravergine) on salads and vegetables. For cooking, in addition to olive oil, oil from seeds, butter, margarine and lard are also utilized. The fats differ in the chemical characteristics of the elements they are composed of, and for this reason, some are suited to accompanying foods while others are better for frying.

Fats should not be seen as something horrifying. They are deposited in the body and form an energy reserve, and are indispensable for absorbing liposoluble vitamins, A, D, E, K, for producing hormones and for the synthesis of bile.

Another fundamental group of nutrients are *vitamins* and *minerals*, which, although they do not provide any energy or supply any plastic material, are essential for the biochemical processes of the living organism to function properly. Fruit and vegetables contain the right quantities needed to fulfill our daily requirements.

Vitamins

Vitamins are necessary only in small doses, and must be present in the food we eat, because our bodies are not able to produce them. They do not represent a source of energy but are indispensable for growth and our vital functions. Vitamins are divided in two categories— *liposolubles,* i.e. soluble in fat (vitamins A, D, E, K), which are transported by lipids, and can thus be stored by the human body, and *water-solubles,* which tend to dissolve in water and can therefore not be stored in the organism, but must be assimilated daily in foods *(vitamins of the B group, vitamin C, folic acid, niacin).*

Amongst the principal vitamins, we point out:

Caption pg. 33

HOW MUCH FAT?

According to the WHO (World Health Organization) fats should represent 30% of our daily calorie intake, of this percentage, less than 10% should be saturated fatty acids.

VITAMIN A (RETINENE). It comes from *carotene,* which is liposoluble, and is transformed into a vitamin in the intestines. It is essential for delaying the aging process, because it is an antioxidant, i.e. acts against free radicals, which are responsible for tumors and for aging. When this vitamin is lacking, the skin becomes wrinkly and dry, and there may be signs of aging and dermatitis on the skin. Moreover, vitamin A is also recommended for defects of vision characterized by reduced visual capacity in faint light or at night *(nyctalopia).*

It is found in carrots and in most green and yellow vegetables, in liver and codliver oil, eggs, milk and dairy products.

VITAMIN B COMPLEX. These vitamins help fight against stress and nervous exhaustion. They are necessary in the event of a prolonged use of medication, such as antibiotics, in case of fatigue, alcoholism, and diets in which an overabundance of refined foods are consumed to the detriment of other fundamental nutrients, such as vegetables and meat. In this group, the most important ones include:

VITAMIN B1 (THIAMINE). Is useful in the event of a lack of energy, chronic fatigue, irritability, and depression; it also helps in fighting against daily stress. It can help those who suffer from nightmares. a symptom that indicates neurological disorders, which this vitamin can reduce, is a tingling or burning sensation in the fingers. In addition to affecting the nervous system, a lack of this vitamin may induce disorders in the functioning of the heart and intestines.

It is found in whole grains, in bread, pasta, yeast and in pork.

VITAMIN B2 (RIBOFLAVIN). Helps release energy from foods and promotes healthy skin and eyes. A deficiency of this vitamin can lead to redness of the eyes, conjunctivitis and cataracts, in addition to inflammation of the tongue. The skin around the nose and cheeks may appear scaly, and ulcerations may form at the corners of the mouth.

It is found in brewer's yeast, milk, meat, liver and in green vegetables.

VITAMIN B5 (PANTOTHENIC ACID). Is useful for metabolizing proteins, fats and carbohydrates, for the production of hormones and protection of the skin, hair and nervous system. A deficiency may cause seborrhoea.

It is found in yeast, whole grains, liver, egg yolks, legumes, fish, nuts and green vegetables.

VITAMIN B6 (PYRIDOXINE). Is needed for metabolizing foods, particularly proteins, and for synthesizing DNA and RNA.

It promotes the production of red blood cells. A deficiency may cause skin damage.

It is contained in cereals, soy flour, meat, liver and legumes.

VITAMIN B12 (CYANOCOBALAMIN). Is needed to protect against pernicious anemia, to maintain normal neural function and for growth.

A deficiency may cause damage to the nervous system, leading to tingling in the fingers and even to severe damage to the nerves, if the material that surrounds them starts to degenerate. This may lead to apathy, mood swings and disorders, paranoia, and, in the most severe cases, to weakness, stuttering and tremors.

This vitamin is found in meat, fish, milk and shellfish.

FOLIC ACID. Is used in the synthesis of nucleic acids and the production of red blood cells. A deficiency of this substance may lead to anemia.

It is found mainly in wheat germ, yeast, green vegetables (cabbage, spinach), in turnips, bran, liver and kidneys.

VITAMIN C (ASCORBIC ACID). Is an antioxidant and antitoxin. It increases the defenses of the organism against infections, lends greater resistance to the lining of the blood vessels, the bones and teeth, and aids in the absorption of iron. It also contributes to producing collagen. A deficiency can cause scurvy, bleeding of the gums, and cracked skin.

It is found in citrus fruits, kiwis, peppers, tomatoes, and even in milk.

VITAMIN D (CALCIFEROL). Is essential for normal growth and teeth formation, since it enables calcium to be absorbed by the bones. A deficiency can lead to rickets in small children and to a serious fragility of the bones in adults (osteomalacia).

This vitamin is found in milk, butter, eggs, cod-liver oil, and tuna fish, and is synthesized as a result of exposure to light rays.

VITAMIN E (TOCOPHEROL). Is, like vitamin A, an antioxidant, that protects the cells of the body from free radicals and from the aging process, Moreover, it increases the fluidity of the blood and is very useful in legs made heavy and tired by poor circulation. Vitamin E stimulates the immune system and helps maintain the proper functioning of the heart and muscles. A deficiency may lead to a dysfunctional metabolism.

It is found in green leafy vegetables, wheat germ, olive oil, vegetable oils, eggs and liver.

VITAMIN K. Is essential for the proper coagulation of the blood and to fight against hemorrhages.

It is contained in liver, soy beans, green leafy vegetables (broccoli, Savoy lettuce, cabbage), and in milk.

VITAMIN PP (NIACIN). Has an important role in the metabolism of sugars, and is used for reactions that release energy. A deficiency may cause dermatitis and a characteristic illness, called pellagra. It is found in meat, fish, yeast, bran and in vegetables.

Minerals

Minerals are substances found in all foods, in differing amounts. They are essential, because they ensure the proper functioning of vital cell processes at all levels of the organism.

Amongst the most important minerals found in the human body in considerable quantities (about 4% of the body weight is, on average, composed of these substances), we find calcium, phosphorus, potassium, and to a lesser extent iron, magnesium and sodium.

Trace elements, on the other hand, are those minerals of which only traces are found in the organism, although they are just as important (copper, zinc, selenium, cadmium, manganese and chrome).

CALCIUM (CA). Strengthens bones and teeth, helps the coagulation of the blood and cardiac contraction, in addition to ensuring the proper conduction of nervous impulses and muscle growth. A deficiency of this mineral can cause rickets and stress.

It is found in milk and its derivatives, green leafy vegetables, dried legumes and in sardines.

PHOSPHORUS (P). Is useful for the proper functioning of the nervous system and al body tissues, in addition to the formation of the bones and teeth. A deficiency can cause poor concentration.

It is found in fish, legumes, meat, milk and its derivatives and in dried fruit.

POTASSIUM (K). This mineral is useful for regulating neuromuscular activity, cardiac function and for stimulating the activity of the kidneys. Furthermore, it helps preserve the liquid in cells. A deficiency may cause cramps and muscular weakness, depression, low blood pressure and tachycardia.

It is found in dried fruit and legumes, and in fresh fruits and vegetables.

IRON Fe. Is found in the red blood cells as a component of hemoglobin. It is useful in preventing anemia and reinforces the immune system of the organism. A deficiency in iron is seen especially in women during their menstrual cycle and may lead to depression, and physical and psychological tiredness.

It is found in liver, meat, green leafy vegetables (spinach), legumes, cereals and dried fruit.

MAGNESIUM (Mg). Is essential for the nervous system to function properly and to assist the cardiac contractions, and is required for many chemical reactions. It is used to attenuate premenstrual discomfort.

Between ovulation and the menstrual period, women require a greater quantity of magnesium, and this is why they are recommended to eat more foods containing it. A deficiency may lead to asthenia and nervousness.

It is found in green leafy vegetables, whole grain cereals, milk, dried fruit and in legumes.

SODIUM (Na). This mineral is necessary for the functioning of the nerves, regulates the exchange of fluids in the body, and proper muscle function. While an excess of sodium may cause liquids to accumulate and lead to interstitial edema, a deficiency may give rise to nausea, muscle cramps, apathy and low blood pressure.

It is found in almost all foods, except fruit.

Natural supplements

To maintain good nutrition, all the nutritive elements required for the organism to function properly must be eaten daily.

Unfortunately, due to the methods of growing food and raising livestock, and then to the preparation and conservation of foods, the nutritional value of the foods we eat is diminished.

This is why it is often necessary, especially when following a low-calorie diet, to complement one's diet with natural supplements that can add a considerable amount of certain substances, particularly vitamins and minerals, that are important to achieve a proper metabolic balance.

Below, you will find a list of a few of the main natural supplements:

BIOFLAVONOIDS. Are found in the cellulose of citrus fruits, in the white part underneath the peel.

They have an effect on the lining of the capillaries and blood vessels, increasing their resistance, and they permit interstitial liquid to be reabsorbed properly in the event of cellulite.

They also have an antioxidant effect, since they fight against free *radicals,* which are responsible for aging. They are also used for premenstrual discomfort, to reduce pain in the breasts, and they reduce bloatedness in the lower limbs.

These elements are often found in nature together with vitamin C, whose properties are further enhanced by them. This is why fruit is always recommended when women have cellulite deposits. When these two substances work together, they appear more effective against fragile capillaries than laboratory synthesized vitamin C alone.

MILK ENZYMES. The non-scientific name to designate unicellular microorganisms that cause fermentation. These bacteria are useful for reestablishing the natural balance in the intestines. In particular, *Lactobacillus acidophilus,* normally found in human intestines, is able to counteract intestinal bacteria that are harmful to health and to reduce the decay process that cause a greater amount of toxins to be absorbed by the body. This bacteria may be less present in cases of dysentery or when antibiotics are taken.

Milk enzymes may also be recommended for individuals suffering from constipation, meteorism and abdominal pain.

BEER YEAST. Is considered the main source of vitamins of the B group, and is therefore recommended for people who have a deficiency of these substances. It helps fight against stress, colitis, constipation, and is useful in cases of diabetes.

WHEAT GERM OIL. This oil has a considerable amount of vitamin E, antioxidant and anti-aging substances. It is useful for fighting against circulatory problems and states of fatigue.

Caption pg. 39

THE GREAT ENEMIES OF OUR HEALTH

Free radicals are highly reactive chemical particles that have lost one electron and that, in order to regain a stable configuration and recover the missing electron, combine with other molecules, thus damaging them (oxidation); in fact, they attack the cells in our organism, causing damage even to the DNA (deoxyribonucleic acid which is found in the nucleus of the cells and contains our genetic make-up). Free radicals are probably the most responsible for aging, cancer, heart disease, alterations in the immune system and in the central nervous system.

They are caused by pollution, cigarette smoke and by sunlight, in addition to poor nutrition. They also form as a result of a bacterial infection, but in this case they have a protective role, since they fight against the pathogenic agent.

Below, you will find a list of a few of the main natural supplements:

BIOFLAVONOIDS. Are found in the cellulose of citrus fruits, in the white part underneath the peel.

They have an effect on the lining of the capillaries and blood vessels, increasing their resistance, and they permit interstitial liquid to be reabsorbed properly in the event of cellulite.

They also have an antioxidant effect, since they fight against free radicals, which are responsible for aging. They are also used for premenstrual discomfort, to reduce pain in the breasts, and they reduce bloatedness in the lower limbs.

These elements are often found in nature together with vitamin C, whose properties are further enhanced by them. This is why fruit is always recommended when women have cellulite deposits. When these two substances work together, they appear more effective against fragile capillaries than laboratory synthesized vitamin C alone.

MILK ENZYMES. The non-scientific name to designate unicellular microorganisms that cause fermentation. These bacteria are useful for reestablishing the natural balance in the intestines. In particular, *Lactobacillus* acidophilus, normally found in human intestines, is able to counteract intestinal bacteria that are harmful to health and to reduce the decay process that cause a greater amount of toxins to be absorbed by the body. This bacteria may be less present in cases of dysentery or when antibiotics are taken.

Milk enzymes may also be recommended for individuals suffering from constipation, meteorism and abdominal pain.

BEER YEAST. Is considered the main source of vitamins of the B group, and is therefore recommended for people who have a deficiency of these substances. It helps fight against stress, colitis, constipation, and is useful in cases of diabetes.

WHEAT GERM OIL. This oil has a considerable amount of vitamin E, antioxidant and anti-aging substances. It is useful for fighting against circulatory problems and states of fatigue.

Caption pg. 39

THE GREAT ENEMIES OF OUR HEALTH

Free radicals are highly reactive chemical particles that have lost one electron and that, in order to regain a stable configuration and recover the missing electron, combine with other molecules, thus damaging them (oxidation), in fact, they attack the cells in our organism, causing damage even to the DNA (deoxyribonucleic acid which is found in the nucleus of the cells and contains our genetic make-up). Free radicals are probably the most responsible for aging, cancer, heart disease, alterations in the immune system and in the central nervous system.

They are caused by pollution, cigarette smoke and by sunlight, in addition to poor nutrition. They also form as a result of a bacterial infection, but in this case they have a protective role, since they fight against the pathogenic agent.

Foods

In order to assimilate all the principal nutrients required by the organism, it is important that our diet be varied, because in nature there is no single food which can meet all the nutritional requirements of our body.

In our daily diet there are some foods that are seldom used, either because they require longer preparation time (1-3 hours) or because of inadequate knowledge about their nutritional value.

Below, you will find a description of the main food groups, which should never be missing from a well balanced diet, even in the event of a problem of excess weight. In this case it is important to follow carefully the advice of your dietologist.

Meat

Meats are divided into white, red and dark meats.

WHITE MEATS. Include meat from kid, lamb, veal, chicken, turkey and rabbit (in addition to fish). They are not sinewy, contain almost no fat and are the most easily digested.

RED MEATS. Include beef, mutton, horse meat, pigeon, pheasant and duck. They are bloodier and therefore more rich in iron.

DARK MEATS. Include all wild game.

Meat, since it is rich in protein, requires less time to digest if it is cooked with low heat. On the contrary, when cooked over high heat, the chemical structure of the protein in the meat is modified, making it tougher and more difficult to digest.

In terms of its chemical composition, meat contains protein, lipids, Minerals (1% iron, potassium and phosphorus), vitamins and water.

The water content may vary between 60 and 80%. Where the water content in the tissues is lower, it is replaced by fat.

Proteins are essential to build and maintain muscles. Inside the cells of muscle tissue, there are nucleoproteins called 'extractive substances' because they can be extracted from the meat with boiling water, as occurs with the preparation of broth. These substances constitute 2.2% of the total and include creatine, creatinine, xanthine and urea.

100 gr. of lean beef contain about 127 Calories, while fattier beef contains as much as 300 Calories. The protein content varies from 16 gr. if the meat is fatty to 20 gr. if it is lean.

Fish

Has a high protein content, though lower in freshwater fish. The lipid content varies greatly from one kind to another. Fish is rich in polyunsaturated fats, which are necessary to defend against the process of arteriosclerosis.

Mushrooms

They contain glucides, very little fat, a lot of protein, water (90%) a small amount of fiber and are very low in calories (15 calories per 100 gr.). About 40% of the protein in mushrooms consists of myosin, which cannot be assimilated by the human organism.

Cereals

Cereals are the main source of energy because of their high carbohydrate content. They also provide protein (gluten, a substance that forms when flour is mixed with water), fiber (cellulose), vitamins (B complex) and minerals, all substances, however, that are contained especially in unsifted whole grain flour.

In the cereal group, the most important ones are:

OATS. Rich in protein and polyunsaturated fat, it has a diuretic effect and appears to cure sterility. Rolled oats can be eaten with milk for breakfast.

WHEAT. Comes in two kinds, soft *wheat* used to make bread and pastries, and *hard wheat* used for pasta. It contains protein, composed of gluten. The grain of whole wheat, along with protein, is also rich in vitamins and oils.

BUCKWHEAT. Very nutritious, it is rich in minerals (Fe), and has all the vitamins of the B complex. It is used to make polenta and cookies.

CORN OR MAIZE. Has a moderate amount of fiber and is used to make polenta (corn mush). It does not contain any gluten.

BARLEY. Along with rice, it is one of the best sources of carbohydrates (approximately 84%) and it contains some fiber. It is used mostly to prepare soups.

RICE. Like corn, it does not contain any gluten, and it is very rich in carbohydrates (about 87%). It is used for risotto, soups, and to make sweets. Unprocessed whole rice is highly nutritious and maintains all of its mineral and vitamin content.

RYE. Contains protein and a fair amount of carbohydrates (about 76%). Rye flour, with its low gluten content, is used to make dark, tasty bread.

Vegetables

They contain mostly water (about 85%), vitamins (especially A and C), minerals and dietary fiber, especially when eaten raw. They help us feel full and are very low in calories.

The best way to prepare vegetables is to steam them or cook them on the grill. In this way their vitamins and minerals are not lost completely.

Legumes

Beans, lentils, chickpeas, broad beans, peas, and soybeans are very highcalorie foods (300 Calories for 100 gr. of dried legumes, 100 Calories for 100 gr. of fresh legumes) and they have a considerable amount of starch and protein, and a fair amount of iron, magnesium, calcium and potassium, in addition to supplying a good quantity of B complex vitamins.

They contain all the essential amino acids with the exception of the sulphurated amino acids (cysteine and methionine, the latter being an essential amino acid). These are found abundantly in cereals and therefore, in order to ensure a diet with a high biological value, it is advisable to eat legumes and cereals together (pasta and beans, pasta and chickpeas, rice with peas, polenta and lentils). Their right proportions are 1 to 3, for example 30 gr. of beans for 90 gr. of pasta.

Soybeans come in red, yellow and green varieties. They have a high protein content (about 40%), compared to that of other legumes (20%), are rich in carbohydrates and lipids, and also have the ability to reduce cholesterol. They are used to produce oil.

Soybeans can be used to prepare 'vegetarian burgers', which are rich in vitamins and minerals.

Soybean lecithin acts as a tonic for the brain.

Fruit

Is rich in water, fiber, vitamins, minerals and sugars such as fructose and saccharose. Fruit (and vegetables) of yellow-orange color (apricot, melon, carrot, peppers) are rich in carotene (vitamin A), while citrus fruits and kiwis are particularly rich in vitamin C. The energy contained in fresh fruit ranges between 35 and 50 Calories per 100 gr., apart from some exceptions (banana, grapes).

Oleiferous fruit (walnuts, almonds, pistachios), on the other hand, contains many Calories (about 500 for every 100 gr.), while farinaceous fruits (chestnuts and dates) have about 200.

It is better to eat fruit in between meals since its fermentation in the intestines may aggravate the problem of bloatedness.

Eggs

Constitute a very important food, because they contain noble proteins, vitamins (A, B2, B12, D and E), minerals (iron) and protective substances for the liver (choline and methionine).

They are not recommended for people who suffer from bile stones since they can cause contractions of the gall bladder. They are rich in cholesterol (about 500 mg per 100 gr.). The recommended amount is three eggs per week.

Dairy products

Milk is a complete food. The kind most used is from cows. cow milk and its derivatives supply above all proteins with a high biological value, in addition to fat, minerals (calcium and phosphorus) and vitamins (A, B, D).

MILK. Contains 3 gr. of protein per 100 gr., sugars (lactose) and easily assimilated lipids. It provides almost all the basic elements required for sound nutrition, calcium and vitamin B12.

YOGURT. Is obtained by the fermentation of milk by the addition of two kinds of bacteria: *Lactobacillus bulgaris* and Streptococcus thermophilus. These cause the lactose to acidify and the casein (milk protein) to flocculate. Its nutritional value is similar to that of milk.

CHEESE. Fresh cheeses have less calories than aged cheese, which, instead, proportionally offers a greater amount of protein.

All kinds of cheese contain proteins of a high biological value, lipids and calcium, while the lactose and vitamins of the B complex are eliminated during the curdling process.

Alcoholic beverages

The main effect these drinks have is due especially to the ethyl alcohol contained in them. This has no nutritional value, but supplies a lot of useless Calories. It is absorbed and utilized rapidly by the body, after being metabolized in the liver, and its assimilation requires no particular digestive processes. It has an energy equivalent of 7 Cal/gr. One glass of whisky contains about 120 Calories, a quarter of a liter of wine about 180 Calories. It is not recommended since it alters the psycho-physical capacity, even though a glass of wine with dinner is allowed, since it stimulates digestion and seems to have a role in preventing vascular diseases.

It is mainly metabolized by the liver (about 80%), and an excessive amount causes damage to this organ as well as to the central nervous system.

When more than 500 ml of alcohol is consumed daily, it can lead to liver disorders, steatosis and, in cases of severe chronic alcoholism, cirrhosis of the liver.

Diet

Food is a necessity. It is the only source of energy that can keep our organism alive, enabling the organs and tissues in our body to function properly. Unfortunately, nowadays in highly industrialized countries, a paradoxical situation exists. On the one hand wealth and prosperity seem to lead inevitably to the increasing consumption of tasty and high-calorie foods, on the other hand, the feminine ideal of beauty is increasingly identified, and communicated by the mass media, with the exalted idea of perfect slenderness, images of almost skeleton-like models, with a tendency toward anorexia.

When someone decides to lose weight because of a problem with excess weight, they must accept the idea that, when the amount of calories consumed is greater than the amount required by a given individual, then they will also gain weight. What regulates this process of transforming food into energy is the *base metabolism*, meaning the amount of Calories required to maintain the vital functions of the organism (keep the heart beating, the other organs working, preserve an even body temperature…) which is measured when the individual is

---

FOODS AND THEIR CALORIES

Group containing from 10 to 30 Calories pet, 100 gr.
All vegetables (except legumes)

Group Containing from 30 to 90 Calories per 100 gr.
Fruit

Group containing from 40 to 100 Calories per 100 gr.
Fish without skin, lean meat. Milk, yogurt One spoon of oil (90 Cal.)

Group containing from 100 to 250 Calories per 100 gr.
Light or low-calorie cheese, not aged

Group containing from 260 to 400 Calories per 100 gr.
Pasta, bread. Cheese. Meat with fat. Pastries

The quantity required for women to maintain their weight with light activity is 2,600 Calories per day, while men require 2,900 Calories.

Caption pg. 46

FAT, AN ENERGY RESERVE

Adipose tissue is essential to the organism, since it constitutes a reserve in the event of food shortages.

awake and in a state of rest from a physical, digestive and emotional standpoint. The *functional metabolism* includes the energy consumed for the base metabolism plus the Calories needed to carry out one's various daily activities (reading, ironing, walking and running).

By calculating the Calories we consume, enables us to recognize whether we have eaten too much compared to what is actually required by the body to maintain its weight. The table we showed on the previous page makes it easier to calculate your daily calorie requirement.

It is a biochemical law. What we put in is what we burn up. The energy we receive from food is utilized by our body to keep it alive. When our body moves more energy must be consumed.

There exist some endocrinological illnesses, such as non-insulin-dependent diabetes, hypothyroidism, Cushing syndrome and Turner syndrome, in which the tendency to gain weight is pathological, but most cases of excess weight are not connected in any way to pathologies and are merely a result of excess Calories.

To better understand the metabolism of lipids, i.e. the way in which they are stored and broken down, I will try to provide some information about the metabolism of triglycerides (fats in food and fat deposited in the tissue), cholesterol and their metabolized products.

The situations in which lipids are mobilized from the adipose tissue include food deprivation, exposure to cold and non-compensated diabetes.

In certain situations of stress, the sympathetic nervous system affects the fat bodies, triggering a reaction in which the fat is dissolved **(lipolysis)** and releasing the fatty acids.

There are certain hormones which trigger lipolysis. They can have a rapid, direct or indirect action, causing the lipolysis of other hormones (ACTH, TSH, Glucagon, Glycocorticoids, or GH—*growth hormone*).

Others inhibit lipolysis, such as *prostaglandin*.

Still others trigger the formation of fat *(lipogenesis)*, such as *insulin*, which helps glucose penetrate into the peripheral tissue. In adipose tissue sugar is transformed into fat deposits.

Caption pg. 47

DIET AND DIABETES

Diabetics should not exclude complex carbohydrates (bread, pasta, rice and potatoes) from their daily diet, since these foods provide an important amount of energy, but simply limit the very rapidly absorbed kinds (monosaccharides) and be very careful with the rapidly absorbed ones (disaccharides). If carbohydrates are excluded, more fats and proteins will be eaten, thus causing an unbalanced diet.

When the metabolic processes of the lipids are altered as a result of unbalanced eating, some pathologies may arise which can at times be very serious. One illness connected to eating disorders and to excess weight is *noninsulin-dependent* diabetes. This generally occurs when a person gains weight. In this case, a good diet is sufficient to eliminate the excess kilos and keep the quantity of sugar in the blood (glycemia) in check.

Another metabolic alteration occurs when blood tests show an increase in the number of lipids in the liver—triglycerides and cholesterol (hyperlipidemia). This increase appears to be associated with a predisposition to arteriosclerosis.

People who are overweight need a change of diet. There are severe forms, often hereditary, where the changes in diet are always accompanied by treatment with medication. In the less severe cases, reducing the calorie intake by following a diet may diminish or normalize the cholesterol concentration levels in the blood. These may be associated with abnormal levels of LDL lipoproteins (the 'bad' cholesterol), the fraction of cholesterol that causes most damage to the blood vessels, that tend to increase with a diet rich in saturated fats—found in meat, butter, entrails and in cheese—and cholesterol (hypercholesterolemia). The HDL, however, are called 'good' cholesterol and are considered to protect against arteriosclerosis. The factors that favor an increase of this cholesterol are physical exercise, estrogen and drinking red wine (one glass per day).

Sometimes even diabetes and hyothyroidism can be associated with hyperlipidemia. In this case the therapy will be aimed firstly at curing the two disorders described in order to obtain indirectly a reduction of cholesterol and triglycerides.

The increase of triglycerides in the blood (hypertriglyceridemia) may be associated with obesity, diabetes, alcohol consumption, kidney failure, lupus disease, oral contraceptives, beta-blockers and with hydrochlorotiazide. High

Caption pg. 48

CHOLESTEROL AND TRIGLYCERIDES

Cholesterol is deposited like arteriosclerotic plaque on the walls of the arteries. For individuals under age 30, the cholesterol in the blood should be reduced to 180 mg/dl and less than 200 mgldl for all adults over age 30.
Triglycerides are the fats produced by the organism from simple carbohydrates (sugar) and alcohol.

triglyceride values in the blood are found in people who have a very high calorie intake, who eat simple carbohydrates and drink alcohol. In this case, it is sufficient to stop eating large portions, reduce sweets and alcoholic beverages.

If after a period of 6 months, the results are not satisfying, a medication suited to each case will be prescribed. Physical exercise can also contribute to normalizing the level of lipids in the blood, which is why people are recommended to walk for at least one hour a day.

The three risk factors that can be acted upon in the event of a genetic predisposition to coronary heart disease are total cholesterol, high blood pressure and smoking. Reducing any one of these factors reduces the risk of arteriosclerosis.

Despite the fact that the risks connected to excessive eating are considerable, nonetheless, for many people, food remains a real 'anxiety outlet', which helps them get by in times of stress and anguish; this makes it even more difficult to have to eat less food. In these cases, in order to achieve noticeable and lasting results, they need to be *educated about good eating habits,* and to analyze their particular situation with the help of a specialized psychologist to gain a better understanding of one's own condition and provides underlying motivations for why they take refuge in food, often to the point of distancing themselves socially from others.

When a person succeeds in following a personalized diet, the needle on the scale will start to move down as much as one kilo per week. At the same time, as I have been able to see in my patients, their self-confidence increases, they experience more positive feelings and their self-control is heightened. Unfortunately, though, if a patient does not learn to eat, at some point they will become tired of the diet imposed by their dietologist and will start eating large quantities of food again, thwarting the results obtained and losing their selfconfidence in their ability to change.

If food is eaten in an excessive manner, without the patient having any possibility of self-control, it is likely that they are suffering from *bulimia.* This disorder is

Caption pg. 49

A proper education on good eating habits as a way to prevent many disorders

characterized by the urge to consume large quantities of food, which is eaten in an uncontrolled manner and repeatedly during the week. Moreover, there may be a need for psychiatric help if the patient, in order to maintain his/her weight, resorts to laxatives, diuretics and self-induced vomiting.

A bulimic person uses food to drown out negative emotions. If they do not have the right food available, they may show symptoms such as a bad mood, tiredness, apathy, a sense of emptiness and tachycardia.

It is better for people who have developed an 'addiction' to certain foods to decide to go on a weight-loss diet during a period when they are not under a lot of psychological stress, either professionally or sentimentally, and they must be highly motivated to lose weight. If not, the increased responsibly from having to follow a diet could aggravate the already existing pressure of the social situation the patient lives in.

Our *eating behavior,* in any case, and especially where there is a 'food addiction', is linked to neurochemical mechanisms. Messages are sent from the brain, which may make us go after a certain quantity rather than quality of food. Once the food is eaten, the brain receives messages of fullness and an *imprinting* for the selection of certain nutrients.

There are many *neurotransmitters*—chemical mediators in the brain that enable electric impulses to be passed from one cell to another—implicated in this mechanism, and they can have various effects:

ADRENALINE. Can stimulate or inhibit hunger according to which hypothalamic receptors (alpha or beta) are stimulated.

NORADRENALINE. When activated it leads to a tendency to eat carbohydrates.

SEROTONIN. Fights against stress, appeases hunger and helps sleep. DOPAMINE. Inhibits hunger.

GABA. Can either stimulate hunger, if it affects the noradrenaline system, or inhibit it, if the serotoninergic system is affected.

Added to these are the neuromodulators:

CHOLECYSTOKININ (CCK). Tends to make us feel full.

ENDORPHINS. May diminish hunger or cause us to choose foods that are rich in protein and fat. Moreover, they reduce stress, improve one's mood, and give a sensation of euphoria; they can also be produced by physical exercise.

These substances may have a particular influence on the choice of carbohydrates and protein, generated by the consumption itself of protein and carbohydrates. Foods rich in sugars, for example, stimulate serotonin. Women generally prefer sweets and all sugary or fatty food, particularly when nearing their menstrual period, due to the effect of the estrogen hormones on the cerebral chemical mediators and on glycemia.

This 'cerebral' need for certain nutrients explains why, in times of crisis, people seek consolation in food, to combat against states of anxiety or depression.

A visit with a dietologist, therefore, will help a person become aware of these unconscious mechanisms, and will enable the patient to learn to eat foods knowing their quality and ideal quantities. Those who want to do things their own way, without seeking help from a specialist, risks making mistakes which could have disastrous consequences. The most common errors are, for example, substituting bread with crackers, or wanting to skip a plate of pasta and lunch and then eating cookies in the afternoon: the consequence of these behaviors may be that the person eats an excessive amount of Calories, without even being aware of it. Seven cookies, in fact, correspond on average to a serving of pasta, just like dressing vegetables—which by themselves are very low calorie—with 4 spoons of oil. Be careful, therefore, about substituting certain foods without the advice of a specialist. In the same way, listening to the advice of a friend who lost

Caption pg. 51

The usefulness of <u>seeing   a dietologist</u>

weight, instead of following a personalized diet, may lead to much confusion.

A diet, as such, does not involve abstinence from certain foods but rather being strict with the amounts of particular foods. It is important to be aware of one's own 'addiction' to certain foods, because this helps us take the necessary measures. For example, those who love chocolate should only keep in the house the amount allowed by their dietologist, eliminating any excess portions. There is no point in substituting that food with another, less-liked one, because they would likely eat both of them.

It has, moreover, been proven that skipping a meal is pointless, because a few hours later we end up eating twice as much. If you are not hungry at mealtimes, there is no need to force yourself. It is better to keep a supply of foods decided in advance, on hand in case of a sudden hunger attack: a can of beans, raw vegetables already washed and chopped, boiled potatoes or a kilo of mixed fruit (apples, pears, citrus fruits). I have been able to observe that the people who manage to reach their goal and do not regain weight easily are the ones who have learned new ways of seeing and behaving with themselves and others.

When, finally, a person loses weight, the subcutaneous fat decreases. If the weight loss is rapid, the skin surface is not able to adapt to the deeper layers, which is why there is a risk of their skin sagging. Weight must be lost gradually, from 500 gr. to 1 kilo per week. The results, naturally, will be varied and will depend on the elasticity of the skin and on physical exercise. When following a diet, it is important to observe your skin to check its elasticity, texture and fragility. If someone has been on a variety of diets, they need to have a more controlled approach, since the food quality and protein calorie balance in particular will play a considerably role. The weight loss may be constant, but some interruptions in the diet will be necessary, during which there will be a stabilization, to give the tissues time to regain their elasticity. Also, after a certain amount of weight is lost, the metabolism tends to slow down, so it is important that the diet be modified to stimulate it again, introducing foods that require more Calories for their own chemical combustion.

Physical exercise is always recommended to burn up more calories and maintain good tone in the tissues. Everyone can give jogging and aerobics a try. I always advise obese people to wait until they have reached their excess weight parameter, because they will find it less difficult to get used to certain kinds of physical exercise. This applies even more for those who have never done much sports before. Moreover, those who wish to begin exercising have to keep their blood pressure under control, because along with the weight loss obtained from a crash diet, there tends to be a drop in blood pressure, and this can cause problems for those already suffering from low blood pressure, since it could weaken the muscles.

Physical exercise should in any case always be carried out with moderation, especially by those not used to it, because when the exercise is prolonged lactic acid forms, which can cause pain and discourage them from exercising.

Problems connected to excess weight and poor eating habits

People who suffer regularly from weight problems, along with the more or less serious trouble caused by possible alterations in metabolism, some problems may arise that are connected to the inadequate functioning of the digestive tract or other organs burdened by the excess weight.

AN IRRITABLE COLON. Is characterized by abdominal pain, meteorism and a chronic alternation of constipation and diarrhea. Nearly 30% of the total population is affected.

Caption pg. 53

THE IMPORTANCE OF MINERALS

It is interesting to know that for every gram of protein synthesized 0.3 gr. of minerals are retained. There are some minerals (magnesium, zinc and sulfur) involved n the synthesis of protein, which help along with physical exercise, the increase of muscle tone. Iron is essential as a component of hemoglobin, necessary for carrying oxygen and carbon dioxide.

Sodium and potassium electrolytes are essential after sports to prevent fatigue and cramps caused by the loss of these elements in the sweat.

It is a disorder in the intestinal motility, aggravated by emotional stress. A particularly sensitive person will be more affected by the emotional tension that can arise in family and job situations.

The abdominal pain comes in the form of cramps, often accompanied by sweaty palms, dizziness, feeling of nausea, anxiety and excessive worrying. It seems to improve with time.

There are a few hygiene and eating habits which can alleviate the symptoms, such as eating regular meals, or cutting down on smoking and coffee. Patients tend, at times, to automatically eliminate some foods which, from their personal experience, seem to cause them trouble.

Often an irritable colon is associated with a deficiency of lactase, enzymes found in the intestines, which are necessary to digest the lactose contained in dairy products (milk, butter, yogurt, cheese, cream, ice-cream, and milk puddings).

When experiencing a period of constipation, it is important to include high-fiber foods in one's diet, such as fruits, vegetables and whole grain foods. Vice versa, when a person has diarrhea these foods should be limited, and they should drink beverages and herbal teas (mint, lemon balm, chamomile and passionflower) with a soothing effect. In more serious cases, it will also be necessary to take tranquilizers. Moreover, milk enzymes are essential to restore the bacterial flora in the intestines.

Those who suffer from such intestinal trouble receive considerable benefits from psychotherapy, analysis and behavioral interpretation, and from exploring their subconscious to understand its repercussions in daily life. This treatment can improve awareness and help adjust to stressful environments. Patients are guided in finding a solution to fears that have deep origins.

METEORISM. Is a disorder characterized by an increased production of gas in the digestive tract. There are foods which foster this situation, and therefore should be avoided, such as dried beans, dried peas, cabbage, radishes, lentils, soybeans, onions, broccoli, cauliflower and cucumbers. In addition, plums, apples, bananas, raisins, whole grain cereals, bran, as well as milk, ice-cream and creams should be limited due to their lactose content. Other guilty parties include fried foods, fatty meats and sauces with butter.

Besides limiting certain foods, however, it is also important to avoid foods and substances that cause air to be swallowed, such as chewing gum. Even whipped cream can make the problem worse.

Also, going to bed right after eating, leading a sedentary lifestyle and stress are all factors involved in creating an excessive amount of gas.

TACHYCARDIA AND ARRHYTHMIA. Additional problems caused by excess weight include tachycardia and arrhythmia, which arise as a consequence of fat that has accumulated in the abdomen, which presses against the heart through the diaphragm (abdominal muscle), causing an irregular heart beat. These tend to disappear once the weight has been lost.

The hazards of unhealthy nutrition are, in any case, always lurking even in those who do not have any specific weight problems. Eating 'impoverished', processed foods, or chemically treated foods may prove damaging to our health if continued over a prolonged period. The enemies of health are lurking almost everywhere. Let us examine a few of the main ones.

Cooking too much meat on the grill, with some burned parts on the meat, and the process of smoking foods, leads to the possible formation of carcinogenic chemical agents, called polycyclical hydrocarbons, and particularly what is known as 3:4 benzopyrene. This is found not only in smoked foods, but also in car exhaust fumes, cigarette smoke and polluted air. If inhaled it can cause lung cancer; if spread over the mucous membranes it leads to the formation of papillomas.

Particular attention should also be given to preservatives: nitrates, inorganic nitrogenous compounds. These are found in cold cuts and canned meats, and in the presence of hydrochloric acid (acid secreted by the stomach which is used for digesting food) are transformed into nitrites and nitrous acid. This can combine with the secondary amines found in protein-based food, and can give

Caption pg. 55

*An unhealthy diet
leads to many problems*

rise to nitrosamines, which are possible causes of cancer.

One disorder that can be caused, in addition to stress, by poor nutrition is *cephalalgia* (headaches). In particular, glutamate (which is found in bouillon cubes) appears to be the subject of criticism following the publication in newspapers of news about a "Chinese restaurant syndrome". People who eat regularly at Chinese restaurants have, in fact, shown a series of symptoms such as headaches and other toxic manifestations. The recommended daily allowance (RDA) is 120 mg per kilogram of body weight. Those who are more sensitive, eating broth every day prepared with bouillon that contains glutamate may prove harmful.

To counteract the various risks brought on by foods that are often not wholesome and by the increasing amount of toxic agents found in our environment, it is important to take antioxidants to combat against free *radicals,* which are also found in the air pollution. Our body has certain defense mechanisms to eliminate some harmful substances, but if there is an excessive amount of such substances, the organism cannot eliminate them all.

There are defense mechanisms that protect against these cell aggressors. They are *antioxidant enzymes,* which stabilize the free radicals. The main antioxidants produced by our body are called: glutation peroxidase, catalasis and superoxide dismutasis.

The antioxidants found in foods include vitamin C, vitamin E, beta carotene and bioflavonoids, which cause the free radicals to become idle. They are found in fruit and vegetables, but can be synthesized artificially. We must nevertheless bear in mind that artificial fertilizers used to grow crops prevent the carotene in uncooked foods, such as carrots and apricots, from being easily converted into vitamin A.

Caption pg. 56

Free radicals
pg. 39

THE BENEFITS OF VITAMINS
Vitamin E blocks peroxidation at the cell membrane level. Vitamin C regenerates the vitamin E and has a direct action against the toxic agents called nitrosamines.

Part Two

A solution to every problem

A study of twelve cases

The case of Giusi

Age 28, h. 168. (h.5,5 feet)

Excess weight: 10 kg=22pounds. Length of treatment: 3 months.

Cm=inch;   h=feet   kg=pounds

	Start of treatment	End of treatment
Weight	kg. 69 =152pound	kg. 59=139ponds
Waist	cm. 79=31,10inch	cm. 73=28,74inch
Hips	cm. 110=43,30inch	cm. 95=37,40inch
Thighs	cm. 64=25,19inch	cm. 55=21,65inch

The case of Raffaella

Age 20, h. 158=5,2

Excess weight: 10 kg=22pounds. Length of treatment: 2 1/2 months.

	Start of treatment	End of
Weight	kg. 57=126pounds	kg. 47=104pounds
Waist	cm. 72=28,34inch	cm. 62=24,4inch
Hips	cm. 98=38,58inch	cm. 92=36,22inch
Thighs	cm. 63=24,80inch	cm. 52=20,47inch
Knees	-	-

The case of Tatiana

Age 45, h. 165=5,4. Vegetarian. Excess weight: 10 kg=22pounds. Length of treatment: 2 months.

	Start of treatment	End of treatment
Weight	kg. 74=163pounds	kg. 64=141pounds
Waist	cm. 73=28,74inch	
Hips	cm. 109=42,9inch	cm. 93=36,6inch
Thighs	cm. 63=24,8inch	cm. 55=21,6inch
Knees	-	-

The case of Elisa

Age 35, h. 161=5,3feet. Has non-insulin-dependent diabetes.

Excess weight: 11.5 kg=25,35pounds. Length of treatment: 3 months.

Start of treatment	End of treatment
Weight kg. 62.5=138pounds	kg. 51=112ponds
Waist cm. 80=31,49inch	cm. 65=25,59inch
Hips cm. 103=40,55inch	cm. 90=35,43inch
Thighs cm. 59=23,22inch	cm. 52=20,47inch
Knees cm. 41=16,14inch	cm. 39=15,35inch

The case of Isa

Age 39, h. 160=5,24feet. Suffers from obesity and an irritable colon.

Excess weight: 18.5 kg=40,87pounds. Length of treatment: 5 months.

Start of treatment	End of treatment
Weight kg. 80. 5=	kg. 62
Waist cm. 95=37,40inch	cm. 75=29,52inch
Hips cm. 119=46,48inch	cm. 99=38,97inch
Thighs cm. 61=24,01inch	cm. 55=21,65inch
Knees cm. 51=20,07inch	cm. 44=17,32inch

The case of Simona

Age 24, h. 176=5,77feet. Suffers from obesity.

Excess weight: 18.5 kg=40,78pounds. Length of treatment: 6 months.

Start of treatment	End of treatment
Weight kg. 83.5=184ponds	kg. 650=143pounds
Waist cm. 85=33,46inch	cm. 63=24,80inch
Hips cm. 118=46,45inch	cm. 95=37;40inch
Thighs cm. 77=30,31inch	cm. 58=22,83inch
Knees cm. 52=20,47inch	cm. 41=16,14inch

The case of Ferri

Age 57, h. 160feet. Suffers from obesity and an irritable colon. Excess weight: 20 kg=44,09pounds. Length of treatment: 6 months.

	Start of treatment	End of treatment
Weight	kg. 85=187pounds	kg. 65=143pounds
Waist	cm. 85=33,46inch	cm. 74=25,13inch
Hips	cm. 102=40,15inch	cm. 95=37,40inch
Thighs	cm. 62=24,40inch	cm. 58=22,83inch
Knees	-	

The case of Raffi

Age 39, h. 165=5,41feet. Suffers from obesity and low blood pressure. Excess weight: 24 kg=52,91. Length of treatment: 7 months.

	Start of treatment	End of treatment
Weigt	kg. 89=196pounds	143pounds=kg.65
Waist	cm. 83=32,67inch	25,19inch=cm.64
Hips	cm. 126=49,60inch	37,40inch=cm. 95
Thighs	cm.75=29,52inch	23,22inch=cm.59
Hips	cm. 126	cm. 95
Thighs	cm. 75	cm. 59
Knees	cm.58	cm. 46

The case of Patrizia

Age 36, h. 160=5,24feet. Suffers from obesity and sideropenic anemia. Excess weight: 29 kg=63,93pounds. Length of treatment: 8 months.

	Start of treatment	End of treatment
Weight	kg. 83=183pounds	119pounds=kg. 54
Waist	cm. 93=36,61inch	25,59inch=cm. 65
Hips	cm. 125=49,21inch	38,97inch=cm. 99
Thighs	cm. 72=28,34inch	22,04inch=cm. 56
Knees	-	-

The case of Valentina

Age 24, h. 159=5,21feet. Suffers from obesity. Excess weight: 30 kg=66pounds. Length of treatment: 9 months.

	Start of treatment	End of treatment
Weight	kg. 86=190pounds	123pounds=kg. 56
Waist	cm. 73=28,74inch	25,59inch=cm. 65
Hips	cm. 112=44,09inch	40,55inch=cm. 103
Thighs	cm. 66=25,98inch	22,53inch=cm. 58
Knees	-	

The case of Caterina

Age 48, h. 162=5,31feet. Suffers from obesity and high blood pressure Excess weight: 29 kg. Length of treatment: 12 months

	Start of treatment	End of treatment
Weight	kg. 94=207pounds	143pounds=kg. 65
Waist	cm. 113=44,48inch	29,52inch =cm. 75
Hips	cm. 121=47,63inch	39,37inch=cm. 100
Thighs	cm. 75=29,52	25,59inch=cm. 65
Knees	–	–

The case of Marinella

Age 31, h. 170. Suffers from obesity and high cholesterol. Excess weight: 50 kg=110pounds. Length of treatment: 18 months

	Start of treatment	End of treatment
Weight	kg.117=258pounds	kg. 67=148pounds
Waist	cm. 125=49,21inch	cm. 75=29,52inch
Hips	cm. 130=51,18inch	cm. 98=38,58inch
Thighs	cm. 78=30,70inch	cm. 55=21,65inch
Knees	–	–

The case of Giusi

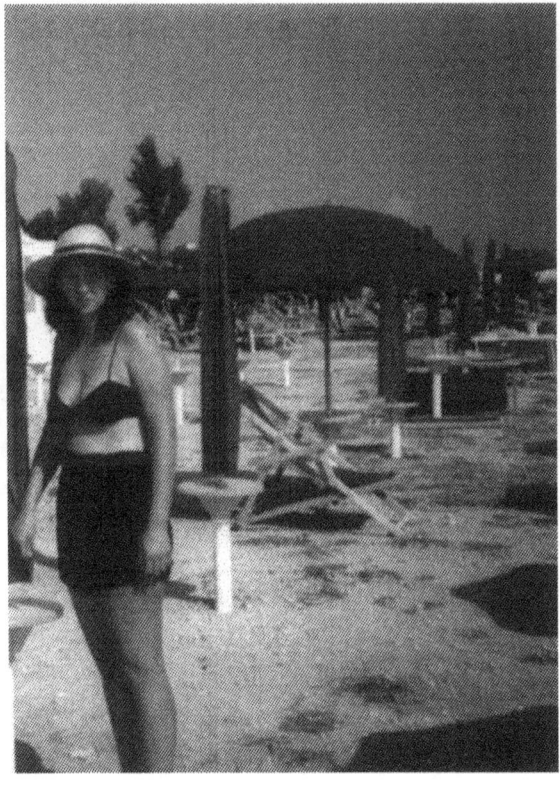

giusy before bw

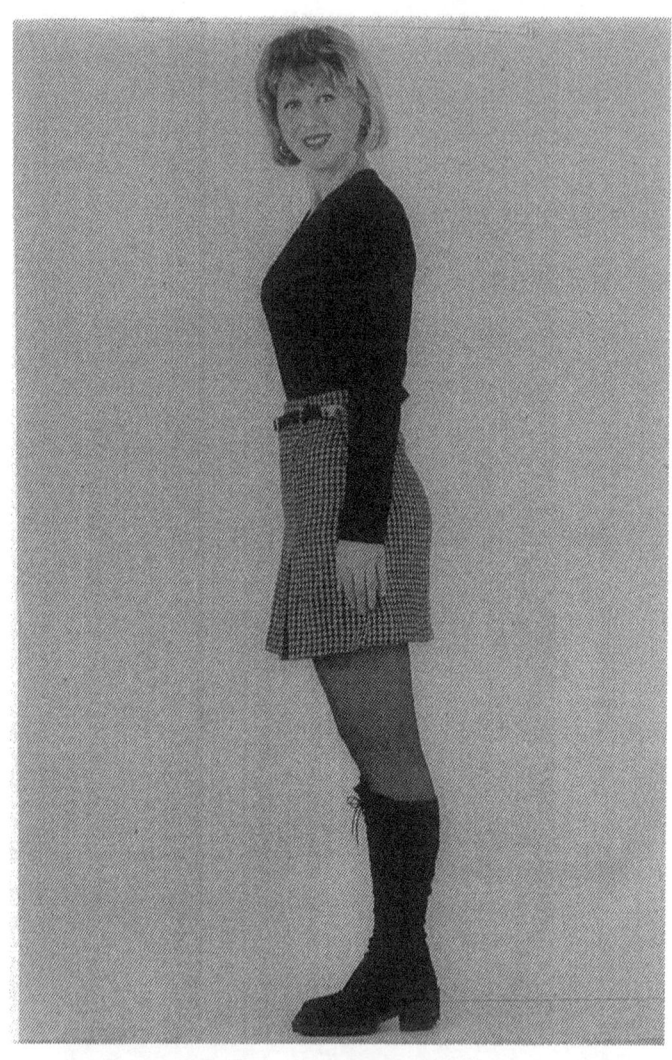

giusy after bw

Giusi was pretty, tall, with red hair, blue-green eyes, an out-going personality, and communicated a certain anxiousness to obtain everything in a hurry.

DIAGNOSIS:

CELLULITE IN THE 4th STAGE, of the flaccid type on the buttocks, edematous cellulite in the trochanter region.

EXCESS WEIGHT: 10 kilos=22lb.

The advanced lipodystrophy (cellulite) in the 4th stage was of the flaccid kind on the buttocks and compact, with ligneous nodules in the upper thigh area. The patient had tried to follow various diets with little success and had used creams.

The first time we met, she told me how she had made the decision to lose weight.

Giusi's motivations

"The desire to seek your help came after a colleague of mine told me how she had lost weight thanks to your help. For me it was essential to receive the guidance of a specialist. By myself I had failed every attempt to lose weight. Psychologically, I am ready this time to make a definite turning point in my life. I want to understand my errors.

For me, being overweight has reached the point of becoming unbearable. I am 28 years old, and I cannot wear what I want. I envy my friends who can show off the latest fashions without any difficulty, while I am always afraid to be conspicuous. My friends and the other girls in the store try to make the problem seem less serious, but I cannot help noticing the two enormous bulging thighs that show so well through my clothes, and which are not only ugly to see, but also painful to the touch. In the past I even went to a beauty surgeon, who advised me to try the only existing remedy at the time: liposuction. I have to admit that I have always had doubts about this kind surgical procedure; a friend of mine, after undergoing liposuction, had the bitter surprise of finding her

Caption pg. 62

LIPOSUCTION

In certain cases this surgical method may be effective but, especially when a large amount of tissue affected by cellulite is removed in a single session, the skin, which no longer has the same support underneath, will show a slackness that is difficult to eliminate with exercise alone. The area treated appears unshapely. Another possible problem may arise when the affected area is emptied of its fatty cushions in an uneven fashion; in this case, the bulges may appear even more accentuated than before.

skin, in the area where the fat had been removed, full of ugly holes. The problems with my figure began when I was 18, and gradually, as time went by, the fat nodules in the upper part of my thighs became large, hard and painful. Despite the fact that my doctor had told me not to worry, the pain was so bad that I could not even sit or lie down on my side. Then the nodules became mountains. I looked at myself with stockings on, but I could not stand seeing my legs in such a state."

WATCHWORD: REACT!

People who find themselves in Giusi's situation experience a veritable internal predicament. They do not accept their own body. Covering their body means avoiding the psychological pain of having to awake to a self-image that they do not admit to themselves. However, even if this strategy might momentarily avert the problem of fat deposits, in the end the seriusness of thir condition will force them to seek out solutions, or they will have to resign themselves to being overweight forever. 80% of women suffer disorders connected to cellulite. Unfortunately, most do not take seriously the risk involved in this disorder, not realizing it can develop into even more serious stages.

"I feel like an unshapely cupboard, I've tried various treatments and have lost a lot of time.

Sometimes I'm afraid there is no therapy suited to my problem and that I will never have any satisfactory results."

I told her this is a common fear for many women, especially if they have made more than three attempts to eliminate the cellulite. They feel discouraged and disheartened by this failure.

"Often my husband points out my problem without any tact, reminding me how fat I am, and this humiliates me because he makes it obvious how useless my efforts to lose weight have been. Sometimes I react, asking him if he loves me or my fat. I seems to me that my body is getting old and less capable of making small efforts. I work in a hotel, walk all day long, go up and down stairs, but even though I move around a lot, the cellulite does not disappear in the least, on the contrary, it has grown worse in these last few years."

I explained to Giusi that in people who are predisposed to it one of the causes of cellulite is a sedentary lifestyle.

"But I move so much, I walk almost eight hours per day! How is it that since I began working, ten years ago, the cellulite has continued to worsen?" Giusi asked me.

Until she was 20 years old, Giusi led a rather sedentary lifestyle; her studies, the tendency to watch TV, her aversion for any kind of sport, taking the pill, very tight jeans and a genetic disposition had worked together and caused the cellulite to develop into the 3rd stage.

It was at this stage that Giusi began working.

The medical treatment

In order to determine the patient's exact weight, I performed an impedenziometry, a technique used to visualize the configuration of the body composition.

I processed the data with a computer to determine the quantity of fat tissue and muscle tissue, in addition to the *base metabolism*.

I concluded that Giusi needed to lose 10 kilos.

Diet

Giusi's usual diet was rich in vegetables and low in fried foods. I made her come back three days later with a daily food chart, in which she had written down all the food she had eaten during the day, and its weight.

She did not get the right amount of protein, meaning meat, eggs and fish. Her buttocks, in fact, hung down (hypotonic) and this emphasized the bulges on her sides. She ate fat cheeses in the evening, but also many sweets, both during the day and late at night, since she did night shifts. Often her meal consisted of sandwiches, usually very thick and covered with mayonese.

When she ate at her work place, she had to bring food from home. I advised the following menu:

Caption pg. 64

NEVER NEGLECT YOUR OWN BODY

It happens quite frequently after they get married for women—but often also men—to have a tendency to neglect themselves. During a conflict, one of the two spouses will often reproach the other for certain flaws (including physical ones). Sometimes these situations can lead to self-criticism and to action. Taking their partner's criticism in a passive manner, without reacting, convincing themselves that there are no solutions to the problem, may instead be very dangerous, because this risks leading them down the tunnel of depression, a state in which one is no longer able to respond to external stimuli, even though it is clear to the person that they need to change. Some women claim to experience their weight problem as a frustration, even in their intimacy with their spouse. They do not feel very desirable, or very sexy. Often it is the person concerned who dramatizes the problem and behaves accordingly, triggering in this way a chain reaction within the couple which leads the overweight person to believe they are not accepted by their partner.

It is not uncommon for couples to rediscover a new closeness once the physical flaw in the wife or the husband has disappeared.

80 grams=3 oz of bread, plus 100 grams3,5 oz of low-fat cheese OR large salad with egg or ham no more than *once a week because very salty OR mixed vegetables. asparagus, broccoli, corn, savoy, radishes and peppers.*

At dinner, instead, she was advised to follow a diet that would include at least the following foods:

300 grams=10,5 oz of fish
AND *70 grams 2 oz of pasta topped with a tomato sauce.*

One day, during the diet she was following, Giusi said something that I like to hear from my patients:

"I have finally learned how to eat, and even at restaurants I don't have any trouble. I follow your advice. If I eat the first course, I try not to finish all the sauce on the pasta, and of course I avoid fried foods.

When I'm eating out, or in case I feel an urge to satisfy my appetite with a large meal, I eat huge portions of grilled fish. If I eat a piece of cake, I do without the first course and bread. I renounce cakes covered with whipped cream or frosting (something I did not do before!), and I opt instead for a bowl of fruit with a scoop of ice-cream, or a piece of pineapple flambè, after having eaten a pasta dish with the restaurant's special sauce. I have maintained my new weight for a whole year now."

During the maintenance period, it was important that Giusi not eat too much bread. Her first (pasta) courses were followed by a second (meat) dish four times a week. The second course consisted of grilled sole or a slice of salmon trout. If, instead, she preferred a large serving of grilled fish, she had to do without the first course. Her diet could include up to about four spoons of oil per day, as much fruit and vegetables as she liked, alcoholic beverages with much moderation, and water, of course, in unlimited quantities.

Caption pg. 65

TOMATO SAUCE

It is easy to prepare, very low-calorie, tastes good and is very filling.
Ingredients:
one can of peeled tomatoes, one envelope of vegetable broth purchased at the super-market, one spoon of bran, plenty of fresh basil.
Combine ingredients and simmer for a few minutes

Internal therapy

To treat her fragile capillaries, the cellulite and swollen legs, I pre-scribed her tablets with *bioflavanoids* and a tincture of *taraxacum*.

Since she had difficulty in feeling a sense of satiety, I prescribed her *ispaghul*.

For the excessive anxiousness about daily problems caused by the job and by the fear of not obtaining results with the medical treatment, I prescribed her a homeopathic preparation, *Sepia compositum*, because it is mixed with other homeopathic products.

For the periodic constipation and to control intestinal function, she had to take, as necessary, *a preparation of fruit fiber and tamarind*.

For abdominal bloatedness, the consequence of eating a meal too quickly, I advised her to eat more slowly and prescribed her an *herbal tea with anise, fennel and cumin* to drink after her main meals.

External therapy

Giusi claimed to have felt a noticeable improvement in her legs already after the first therapy sessions were held.

I carried out a cycle of medical therapies, alternating a series of *mesotherapy* treatments based on drugs to stimulate the blood circulation with *ultrasound therapy* sessions. After four sessions, I also began using *magnetic therapy*. During the final sessions lipolytic drugs were used in combination with the ultrasound therapy.

This therapeutic pattern was followed to restore the circulation, break down the tissue affected by cellulite and dissolve the fat trapped in the fibrous tissue.

I carried out a total of 16 sessions combined two at a time for each session.

Caption pg. 66

HEALING WITH PLANTS

Despite the ever increasing number synthetic drugs, modern pharmacotherapy still draws many active substances from the plant world Medicinal plants and the preparations made from them (infusions, decoctions, extracts…) are widely used for and effective in treating health problems,
pg. 184-93
Mesotherapv pg. 200-01 Ultrasound therapy

pg. 201-03 Magnetic therapy pg. 205-06

The change

At the end of the therapy, Giusi told me the results she had obtained:

"Now I feel in good shape even in the evening. During the day I work twelve hours, eight hours standing and moving around a lot. I try not to remain standing in the same position, as you advised me. I have long and tiring days, but in the evening I still feel like tidying up the house, going out and being with my husband. First, my shirts were size 44, but my pants were at least two sizes bigger. I could not buy close-fitting pants, but only those with pleats, large in the hips, size 48, and I had to pull them in at the waist, while they were tight around my thighs. I realized that it was not enough to just go on a diet, because once I managed to lose four kilos, all in the bosom, while my thighs stayed the same. I was terrorized when you told me I should lose 10 kilos, but I calmed down when you explained the effects the therapy would have."

I thought about how much Giusi had changed, both physically and psychologically.

As her lumps of cellulite disappeared, her skirts became shorter. Giusi continued:

"Finally I can allow myself to wear what I like. Not even when I was 18 did I let myself wear a skirt this long and this straight!"

On her face was an expression of infinite gratitude.

"I feel like revolutionizing everything," she declared "and it looks as if the revolution has already begun."

I did not think Giusi's problem affected her so much, but now, observing her more closely, her hair seemed redder than usual, her haircut more modern. She was wearing a black shirt, a very short yellow skirt, tall black boots, dark stockings. She looked like a model.

Caption pg. 67

*EATING LESS IS **NOT ENOUGH***

Almost all women who are affected by cellulite have tried to go on diets and know that this disorder does not disappear by merely reducing the amount of food they eat.

THE PLEASURE OF BEING ADMIRED

It is interesting to observe how all women, as they gradually get rid of excess weight and bulges, want to be admired by others again. This is due to the fact that they are learning how to like and accept their own body, finally realizing that they've changed. At the psychological level this amounts to a boost of selfconfidence.

"I have found a second job", she announced happily.

Her friend had a clothes store and had asked her to model some of the clothes to induce customers to purchase them.

Giusi added with greater emphasis:

"She claims to sell more this way. You see how satisfying it can be to be thin? My husband now notices the way I dress. He is jealous, and I'm glad about that. I like to be looked at. At work the others joke around and tell me that now they can flirt with me. I answer: 'You couldn't before?' ".

'Plans for the future?' I asked her.

Giusi thought a moment, became serious and answered with a soft voice:

"I'm considering having a baby!".

The case of Raffaella

Raffaella was a lively girl, age 20, with a tendency to exaggerate her own flaws; she came to me, asking me to help her lose weight because she felt too 'plump'.

DIAGNOSIS:

CELLULITE IN THE 2nd STAGE, edematose type. EXCESS WEIGHT: 10 kilos=22 poundsj

CONSTIPATION. Problem over the last years. HYPOPOTASSEMIA (lack of potassium in the blood).

From a clinical point of view, as far as the patient's legs were concerned, the situation was not too serious. The leg area was affected by edamatose cellulite in its second stage, which is easily treated.

This is how Raffaella remembers her situation before treatment.

Raffaella's motivations

"I saw my behind was wide, my hips and knees swollen, and bulges on my thighs as if they were fat. For years my ankles had been sweling up on me, for the past five years I had been waking up in the night with pain in my legs from cramps.

I went on a diet, because I was dissatisfied with myself. I lived waiting for the day when I would be thinner. I was unhappy about everything, including my sentimental life. I had been dating a guy for two years. He like me the way I was, with those extra pounds, but this wasn't good enough for me, I wanted to change everything, to change boyfriend and to change figure.

I was ashamed of my body. I began to lose weight towards the end of our relationship, but he did not want to accept the change in me. He thought I wanted to be prettier so other guys would be attracted by me. In the end, when he left me, he told me that I wasn't attractive to him anymore. 1 realized I needed to learn to know what I really wanted. Before, I would fall into self-pity, thiking that no one liked me, but bottom line I myself did not like how I looked.

Caption pg. 69

CRAMPS

Cramps may be caused by a lack of potassium.

I wore loose clothes to hide my figure, and to me I did not look very feminine or very sexy. Even if I was not extremely fat, I felt uneasy, and this came out in how I behaved, because I was convinced that others were always sizing me up and critisizing me.

I was what would be defined a "happy-go-lucky person", I tried to make the good side of my character stand out, in the hopes that they would appreciate me at least for my good nature, and I was always available for my friends.

I was convinced that guys thought of me as: 'the nice, plump girl' and I feared that I would never be accepted if I didn't change my looks and my character to please others.

My problem is that I did not have a clue about how to lose weight. I had tried to go on diets described in newspapers, but was never able to stick to them. If I did not see concrete results after a week, I gave up.

My mother did not think I would be able to stick to a diet. My parents thought I looked fine even with those extra pounds."

The medical treatment

Diet

Raffaella came to my office determined to follow my advice. She was a student and did not have any trouble following a diet in which the food had to be weighed. She asured me that she already had a little scale and wanted to learn how to follow a personalized diet.

She had trouble with constipation, and very slow intestines, and a diet could aggravate the problem.

I explained to her that this problem arises when we do not have enough vegetables in our diet, so I prescribed her a diet of 1200 Calories that took account of this need, and in which she could eat as many vegetables as she liked.

Caption pg. 70

1200-Calorie diet
pg. 160-63

Her blood tests had revealed a potassium deficiency. Her nutritional casehistory showed a lack of foods containing this element in her diet. I gave her a table of foods that are particularly rich in potassium (see across) and included this factor in her computerized diet.

I advised her the following diet of three days of 1200 Calories with the exact amount of *protein (15%), lipids (30%)* and *carbohydrates (55%)*.

> <u>Day 1</u> BREAKFAST *1 fresh squeezed orange 50 gr=2 oz whole wheat bread+1 slice cheese and one slice of ham*
> LUNCH *plenty of lettuce+60 gr 2 oz rice+100 gr 3 oz low-cal cheese*
> DINNER *200 gr 6 oz boiled potatoes+150 gr=4,5 oz steamed shrimp+rucola lettuce to taste*
> <u>Day 2</u> BREAKFAST *150 cc 4,5 oz of 2% milk+20 gr 1 oz rolled oat flakes*
> LUNCH *salad with fennel+carrots+60 gr=2 0z spaghetti+plenty of tomato sauce+20 gr=1 oz Parmesan cheese+fruit and low-fat yogurt*
> DINNER *boiled carrots+trout baked in foil+50 gr 2 oz soy bread*
> <u>Day 3</u> BREAKFAST *tea+3 slices of toast*
> LUNCH *one grilled steak+chicory to taste+pack of whole wheat crackers+fruit yogurt*
>
> **DINNER *vegetable soup+50 gr chick peas+raw vegetables+fruit to taste***

The positive thing was that Raffaela liked many of the suggested dishes on the menu.

Following this diet of approximately 1200 Calories for a period of three weeks, with a one-week break every month, so as not to follow an imposed diet, she arrived at her maintenance period after two and a half months. Raffaella ended her dietary treatment a few days before leaving on vacation. She was able to follow her maintenance diet during the summer, without much difficulty.

The Calories required to maintain her weight loss ranged between 1600 and 1800, depending on the amount of physical exercise she did. The amount of potassium contained in her food grew as the calorie intake increased. The introduction of legumes, very rich in potassium and nearly non-existent in her previous diet due to their high calorie content, enable her to spend the summer without any risk of hypopotassemia, because it is normal in the summer to lose greater amounts of this mineral from sweating. Whole grain foods are also rich in this very necessary element.

Raffaella proudly told me what she had achieved:

"I have learned to eat the right way, I have become independent and no longer eat with my parents. We are from the south of Italy. We love very rich dishes and fattening foods. Now, though, I have created my own personality from a nutritional standpoint. I like wholesome, low-fat foods. If I eat a dessert or pasta, I skip the bread. When I slip up, I try to eat less the next time."

Internal therapy

For her chronic constipation, the meteorism (air in the abdominal area) and her abdominal pain I prescribed her milk *enzymes* and an *herbal tea of frangula,*

Caption pg. 72

IN THE SUMMER IT'S EASIER

In the summer, when it's hot, people feel less hungry, and many find it easier to follow a diet to maintain their weight loss.
Phytotheraov pg. 184-93

and I advised her to drink during the day one liter of broth prepared with artichokes, carrots and potatoes (see across).

Raffaella was also taking the *contraceptive pill.* Unfortunately, in many women this causes water retention, which is felt especially in the thighs and legs.

In addition, some 2nd degree cellulite had formed in her legs. In order to eliminate this, it was enough to stop taking the pill for two months.

For her problems linked to water retention, I advised her to take pilosella, taraxacum and *Bermuda* grass three times daily for twenty days a month.

I also prescribed *potassium* supplements to take every other day for two months for her night cramps.

External therapy

Raffaella had cellulite deposits in her legs that were not yet serious and which were reduced with dieting and exercise, even though she retained two side cushions. Therefore, upon her request I opted for medical therapy.

I applied *ultrasound therapy* with the lymphodrairage program for ten minutes, given her predisposition to lymphatic stagnation, and I used local *mesotherapy* for the saddlebags on her thighs. I followed this with twenty minutes of ultrasound therapy.

The change

At the end of the treatment Raffaella told me she finally felt good about herself:

"My cramps have disappeared, I no longer suffer from constipation or colitis, and I often wear mini-skirts. I feel light and am more active. I was used to seeing my face looking run down, now I feel much prettier.

I have reached my goal, am carefree and out-going.

I have tried everything to improve, and now I don't mind if someone doesn't accept me. I am aware of my qualities as well as my weaknesses. I know that is the best I can do.

I have a new boyfriend who met me when I was thin, and he cannot imagine how I was before. After the summer vacation I selected a fashion that showed off my figure. Many of my friends seeing me lose weight thought I was lovesick. Getting rid of those extra pounds has also eliminated my insecurity, now I feel much stronger. My behavior has changed and people have noticed the difference. I am more determined, more aggressive and sometimes, as my friend says, more selfish. Now I prefer to say what 1 think."

Raffaella studied psychology and had a real ability to analyze issues with a professional outlook. I asked for her opinion about the change many women undergo once they have obtained their new figure.

"In my view, women change because they regain confidence in themselves. When you're fat, you see those around you as the cause of all your problems. The more you depend on the approval of others, the more you blame others for your own troubles. I have experienced this personally. Now I'm no longer preoccupied with obtaining approval from others, because I'm at peace and more especially approve of myself."

The case of Tatiana

Tatiana was a 45-year-old woman, concerned about the onset of menopause and absolutely determined to lose weight without however renouncing her vegetarian "beliefs" whatsoever.

DIAGNOSIS:

CELLULITE IN THE 2nd STAGE, edematose type in the ankles. EXCESS WEIGHT: 10 kilos=lb.
VEGETARIAN.

He ankles were affected with edematose cellulite already in the second stage, which had arisen after she had switched to a strict vegetarian diet, with its implied lack of noble proteins and adequate combinations of amino acids, and combined with the water retention caused by the numerous hours she spent standing in one position.

Tatiana told me why she had decided to seek out my assistance.

Tatiana's motivations

"I keep gaining weight, I'm 45 years old and I've gained ten kilos in the past two years. I am approaching *menopause* and do not want to accept becoming a fat lady.

My face and my body have changed, I don't recognize myself anymore. I feel bloated, and even my smile is gone. My stomach shows and my hips are too wide. I cannot close the zipper on my clothes, I feel like I'm hanging out all over the place. I always have that heaviness in my ankles, and some pain when I'm sleeping or sitting.

Whenever I look at myself in the mirror, I think I look awful and, unfortunately, my bad mood affects those in my family too.

I've been a vegetarian for ten years: I don't eat meat, I eat fish only once in a while and I have completely eliminated cheese from my diet. I seldom drink milk and I eat eggs twice a week."

The medical treatment

Diet

From Tatiana's description, I deducted that she was not nourishing herself adequately. She ate a lot of legumes and whole grain foods, but even though these are rich in amino acids, they did not provide her with the right amount of noble proteins.

She did not want to eat meat, since she was against killing animals.

She had eliminated nearly every kind of cheese from her diet, convinced that it was fattening, and she thought that eggs did not have a high nutritional value. On the other hand, she ate unlimited quantities of soy burgers, pasta and whole rice, in addition to legumes, vegetables and fruit.

She told me she was willing to increase the amount of cheese and eggs she ate and to add tunafish to her diet, the only fish she liked.

First of all, I gave her a few general rules she had to follow:

AT LUNCH she could eat cereal, pasta or gnocchi topped with low fat cheese or an egg or meat.

AT DINNER she had to prefer a single course such as pasta and chickpeas, pasta and beans or soy burgers.

I prescribed her therefore a three-day, ovo-lacto vegetarian diet of 1500 Calories, leaving in her favorite foods and adding the correct daily portion of protein. In addition, I drastically reduced the intake of alcoholic beverages, which Tatiana drank excessively.

Day 1 BREAKFAST *corn flakes (2 large spoons)+a cup of partially skimmed milk*

LUNCH *cream of vegetable soup+rolled oats (2 spoons) one egg, raw vegetables*

DINNER *chickpea soup (1 can) with one leek, one clove of garlic and parsley 80 gr 3 oz soy bread one yogurt oil (two spoons a day)*

Day 2 BREAKFAST *Coffee and milk+3 slices of toast*

LUNCH *2 oz of spaghetti with 1 oz clams cooked and raw vegetables one piece of fruit*

DINNER *sole+vegetables fruit oil (2 112 spoons over 24 hours)*

Day 3 BREAKFAST *Tea+2 slices of toast+jam (2 tea-spoons)*

LUNCH *6 oz polenta weighed cooked+100 gr 3 oz low-fat cheese citrus fruit*

DINNER *90 gr 3 oz pasta with 30 gr 1 oz dried beans one yogurt, one piece of fruit oil (1112 spoons over 24 hours)*

Internal therapy

For the swelling caused by water retention, I prescribed taraxacum.

Her abdomen was bloated because of meteorism (air inside the abdomen), the heaviness and sleepiness after meals were symptoms of poor digestion; for this I prescribed her cardo mariano, melissa, luppolo and vite.

Caption pg. 77

Phvtotherapy
pg. 184-93

External therapy

To accelerate the reabsorption of the interstitial liquid and reduce the edema and pain, I gave her five sessions, on a weekly basis, of laser therapy.

The Change

Tatiana told me she was satisfied during one of our last therapy sessions:

"I have not changed my eating habits, I eat the same cereals as before, and I do not make any sacrifices, except perhaps having to eat cheese, which before I had crossed from my diet, along with eggs and fish. I had to force myself to introduce this protein, but I did not feel hungry or desire foods I wasn't allowed to eat. The extraordinary thing is that instead of becoming flabby with the loss of weight, my body is now firmer, and 1 realize that, just as you told me, muscle tone depends on the amount of protein we eat, which I did not get enough of before.

My ankles, which were my main source of worry, have become thinner and, above all, do not hurt any more. In two months I lost ten excess kilos and regained my good mood.

Caption pg. 78

Laser therapy
pg. 204-05

The case of Elisa

Elisa came to me as if I were her last hope. She lived in Tuscany, and to reach me she had to travel 400 kilometers. She considered the trip as a kind of pilgrimage to obtain good health. She told me that I could not disappoint her because she trusted in me.

DIAGNOSIS:

EDEMATOSE CELLULITE. EXCESS WEIGHT: 11.5 kilos 25, 35pounds NOWINSULIWDEPENDENT DIABETES. MAGNESIUM DEFICIENCY.

Her cellulite was of the edematose type, located in the upper thigh area; sclerotic stress, typical of the 3rd stage in the trochanteric area. Probable cause; prolonged hormone treatment.

It was Elisa herself who reminded me, at the end of her treatment, what she had felt in the past.

Elisa's motivations

"One evening I bent over to tie my boots, but I realized what an effort it was for me to do this simple movement. A strong sense of emarassment overcame me, I felt stiff and old, even though I was only 35 years old. It was in that aweful moment that I decided to change my life. That is now all behind me, but I remember well how visible around my thighs the deposits of fat, and the folds and hollows in my skin were. I avoided looking at myself in the mirror, I ran away from the problem because I could not accept myself.

Before losing weight I did my hair and dressed in a way that would me remain anonymous. I didn't realize that even though my situation was bad, I could still have improved it.

I tended to get fatter every day, but I refused to buy larger-sized clothes.

My figure was not proportioned; I wore a size 42 above the hip, and below the hip even a size 46 clung tightly, making my bulges obvious, and despite all this, I refused the idea of having to buy a larger size.

I will always remember the frustration I went through, the more or less concealed dissatisfaction, that I pretended didn't exist. Those who've never had weight problems cannot understand how it feels to try on a skirt that ruthlessly uncovers two fat knees.

It was as though I lived in a state of numbness, and I kept putting off finding a solution to my problems. I tended to be depressed and even more so when my period was about to start. Moreover, on those days I felt more bloated and from one day to the next I gained as much as two kilos."

The medical treatment

Diet

Before coming to me, she had been diagnosed with non-insulin-dependent diabetes. The news had frightened her a great deal, because she knew that if not treated this illness could entail some serious complications.

Her blood tests revealed an increase in her glucose level (glycemia) to 150 mg on an empty stomach. There was a tendency toward diabetes.

After the first month of following her diet, the figures returned to normal levels without any need for medication to reduce her blood sugar (hypoglycemic).

Elisa continued to tell me how she behaved towards this newly diagnosed illness:

"The dietologist told me to follow a special diet, but I decided to do what I wanted. I eliminated pasta, bread and sweets because I wanted to lose weight and at the same time reduce my diabetes., but this didn't happen, and my glycemic levels stayed high."

The first month I prescribed her a 1200-Calorie diet that made her lose four and a half kilos.

Caption pg. 80

1200-Calorie Diet
pg. 160-63

It was absolutely essential for Elisa to understand and follow a balanced diet. Therefore, I suggested a diet with 55% carbohydrates, 30% lipids, and 15% protein. She got enough minerals, in particular magnesium, because they were found in her vegetables, especially the green beans, corn and fresh legumes.

The second month her diet was simplified by eliminating the first course at lunch and leaving in plenty of fish and meat in its place. For dinner, three times a week I recommended a menu having only one main dish: vegetable soups with pasta and beans or pasta and chickpeas, or soya and lentils. Her glycemia had returned to a normal level of 90 mg/dl. With this blood sugar level, she was allowed to have an occasional dessert: as an afternoon snack, therefore, I let her eat a small bar of chocolate. That way she could satisfy her sweet tooth, without feeling too deprived of the things she liked as she followed her dietary program.

After three months Elisa reached her ideal weight.

Internal therapy

For her diabetes I prescribed her olivo and *nettle (Urtica)*.

For her edema (water retained in tissue) in the lower legs I advised her *ash*.

For her premenstrual discomfort I told her to take milfoil and *magnesium* one week before her period.

For the bloatedness in her stomach, I recommended her *thyme*.

External therapy

I suggested to Elisa that every evening at home she do massages with creams containing *horse-chestnut* and *menthol:* the former aids circulation, while the second gives a feeling of freshness.

Its effectiveness is felt when the preparation is applied to tired feet.

Once my patient had reached her ideal weight, she did not feel completely satisfied, because she still had two small cushions showing on her sides. Indeed, I had noticed them myself as she was losing weight, and I had already mentioned that it would be very difficult to get rid of them altogether because of the compact cellulite in its third stage.

Elisa would have been ready to follow my instructions, but since she lived in Toscana, it was impossible for her to do regular sessions at the time. At the end of her diet, however, she found the time for the sessions too.

I opted for the most drastic method, which allowed me to solve the whole problem in just five sessions: mesotherapy with hypotonic solutions, lipolytic drugs, cellophane covering, and maximum strength *ultrasound* therapy for 40 minutes, twice as long as normally used. This way the ultrasound therapy worked in a much more aggressive way; my patient felt some discomfort and later there were some small scabs in the area of the injections.

In order to prevent bleeding and make the wounds heal faster, I then used infrared laser treatment. After five sessions the desired results were achieved.

Exercise

Every day Elisa had to do exercises at home to burn off the fat and cellulite in the more difficult points (legs, hips and abdomen).

The change

Elisa concluded her story highlighting how much she had changed:
"I have learned how to eat. I do not deprive myself of anything, but if one day I overdo it and eat too much, the next day I eat less.

Now I wear a size 42. I am not unproportioned anymore. The swelling in my legs

Caption pg. 82

Mesotherapv pg. 200-01 Ultrasound therapy pg. 201-03
Laser therapy pg. 204-05

pg. 194-97

has gone down, and they are smoother and don't hurt me anymore. My weight is what it used to be years ago, but I have also lost several centimeters in the most difficult areas. To give an example, two years ago, with the same weight as now, this skirt was tight on me and my saddlebag thighs were obvious.

The treatment I underwent has made me feel younger. I get along better with others and myself. My friends are amazed and say that ever since I lost weight, I've become more energetic, instead of always tired like before.

It's true; this newfound energy has also helped me make a turning point in my job. Before 1 kept putting it off month after month, but in the end I made up my mind and left my job. I wanted a job that would give me satisfaction and in which I could create something of my own, and now I've succeeded. I decided to give a fresh boost to my father's shoe factory. Feeling good physically has also affected me psychologically.

My way of relating with others has changed. Now I want to dedicate more time to myself, I can't wait to be in new situations.

Recently, I visited an exhibition abroad where I was able to spend time with a lot of new people, but also people from my country whom I had not seen in a while. It was like passing a test. I felt like I was waking up after a long time from a deep slumber to reap the fruits of this new and satisfying life of mine.

The pleasure of feeling different about myself physically gives me extra zest. Now I lead my life in a much more active manner."

The case of Isa

Isa was a woman, age 39, with a very young looking face. She had long, soft, black hair, delicate facial features and fair skin.

DIAGNOSIS:

MEDIUM OBESITY, ANDROID TYPE.FAT AND CELLULITE located in the inner thighs. EXCESS WEIGHT: 18.5 kilos=40,78 pounds.

IRRITABLE COLON.

This patient had fat located particularly in the abdominal area. The inner thighs affected by adipose tissue and cellulite in its third stage.

Isa wanted to retrace her steps and to get back to a perfect figure, analyzing with a more detached perspective her decision to change.

Isa's motivations

"I decided to go on a diet, because I didn't feel good about myself. I started my days with a sense of anguish, I dressed sloppily, I considered myself ugly, so I was always unhappy and depressed. I did not recognize my psychological and physical state right away. My awkwardness around others, due to my excess weight, increased every day and at the same time I kept gaining more weight.

I had a habit of resorting to food to drown my worries and stress, and the fatter I became, the more I indulged in every sort of binge.

The first time you saw me, I could not even cross my legs. I was extremely clumsy. When I sat down, I didn't know in which position to sit, I always felt ill at ease, but by then I had already decided that by my 40th birthday I would be able to show off my former figure again. I had made the firm decision to lose that weight once and for all.

After my second pregnancy, at age 27, I gained 16 kilos, then I lost four, but soon

THE WAY WE SEE FOOD

At birth, the bond between food and love is formed. A baby cries and his mother feeds him. Food becomes synonymous with comfort and security. The same thing occurs as babies grow up: sweets and other treats are used not only to nourish them, but also to placate their feelings of distress. Thus, it is during childhood that people begin to confuse hunger with emotions connected to painful moments. The child learns that his feelings of sadness and insecurity disappear when mommy shows her affection by giving him a candy. Sometimes we use food to fill our hard times in life.

This pattern is mentioned by nearly all of my patients who have a 'morbid" relationship with food. Indeed, all of them remember having been given sweets

to console them. It is important to learn to recognize those times when the need for comfort becomes urgent, and to analyze one's family background and that of one's companion to determine whether this is not what triggers off this strong emotional need. Depression can increase proportionately with an increase in excess weight, but it also diminishes when the weight is lost. In a married couple, generally when this happens husbands becomes more attentive, because they realize their wife could be attractive to another man.

The key to success lies in becoming aware of how you feel and deciding to take action to change the situation.

started gaining weight again until I finally weighed 81 kilos at age 39. Before going on a diet and undergoing medical treatment, my thighs were suffocating under mountains of cellulite. My waistline and upper body were one big trunk, my breasts were small and covered with fat. If I looked at the floor standing up straight, I could not see my feet. I had respiratory trouble, which got worse whenever I went up a just a few steps; carrying groceries required a huge effort for me. I had to walk slowly and I felt like an old granny.

My husband's muttered comments and his behavior made it obvious, even if he didn't say it so many words, that I was no longer attractive to him and wasn't the girl for him that I used to be. Unfortunately, I believe that people who are pleasing to the eye are treated with greater consideration, regardless of their real worth as a person. Before, if someone paid me a compliment, I realized it was only out of politeness.

When I happened to see an old picture of myself, I would tear it up because I couldn't stand seeing the sight of myself so different.

Caption pg. 85

THAT'S NOT REALLY ME

In cases where a weight gain has caused a considerable change in someone's appearance, they may even go so far as to deny the change or not recognize themselves.

My children helped me stick to my diet, checking on me constantly. Sometimes to put my will power to the test they would eat an ice-cream in front of me, reminding me with a mischievous look that I could not even have a taste.

I realized that I had really decided to take my diet seriously, with my mind, not just with my words. Psychologically, I was ready and determined to go all the way.

At the office people noticed the changes in me and they complimented me on my new way of dressing, for my good mood and younger looking appearance. This made me feel so proud and encouraged me to not let go of my goal."

THE APPROVAL OF OTHERS IS THE BOOST TO CONTINUE

The apathy felt by those who are struggling with their inability to make a concrete decision to lose weight once and for all tends to vanish like magic once definite action is finally taken. Suddenly we are not alone anymore, for we realize that others notice the change in us too. This reduces stress, because compliments relieve anxiety more effectively than food. They represent the approval and esteem of others, both of which are necessary to live happily in society. Our self-esteem, moreover, consequently increases. This could be described by a phrase that my patients often repeat when losing weight. '! can do it'.

The medical treatment

Diet

Isa suffered much as a result of her physical appearance, but by herself she was incapable of losing weight. For her it was essential to follow a balanced, 1200-Calorie diet that made her lose one kilo a week.

The fact that she was so determined helped her, even when she was tempted to transgress, to visualize the pain induced by her condition.

She confessed to me that in the beginning she missed the butter rolls and chocolate, but with her willpower she was able to overcome the temptation to eat them. The, gradually, her urge for sweets disappeared.

I set her some goals that were easy to reach and a diet rich in fiber found in

Caption pg. 61

1200-Calorie diet
pg. 160-63

vegetables; in addition, to reduce her feelings of hunger I prescribed her some plant-based products.

AT LUNCH she ate at the cafeteria wheel she could not weigh her food. I told her to eat grilled meat or fish. Since the cooks added quite a bit of oil, and thus the amount of Calories increased, she had to use a teaspoon for her salad dressing. She could eat as many raw vegetables as she wanted, as long as she didn't add more than two teaspoons of oil. She was allowed to eat mozzarella twice a week, tunafish and ham once a week. No bread, breadsticks or crackers. No pasta or rice dishes, because it wasn't possible to determine exactly how large the portions were.

AT DINNER I prescribed her instead a diet in which it was necessary to weigh her food: since she had to cook for her family, she avoided the bother of having to cook separate dishes.

> 60 gr=2 oz pasta weighed before
> cooking OR 120 gr=3 oz cooked
> pasta OR 60 gr=2 oz rice weighed
> before cooking OR 120 gr 4 oz
> cooked rice OR 80 gr 2,5 oz whole
> wheat bread OR 200 gr=5 oz

potatoes OR 200 gr=5 oz cooked
polenta OR 200 gr=5 oz gnocchi
+
100 gr=3 oz meat
OR 250 gr=4 oz
cooked fish
OR 70 gr=2 oz
mozzarella
OR 50 gr=2 oz
cured ham OR
two boiled eggs

SATURDAYS AND SUNDAYS, since she ate at home, she had to follow a menu of her choice from those suggested for her evening meals.

This diet remained unchanged for two and a half months, and at the end of this period she ceased to lose weight. For Isa it had become difficult to be on the imposed diet, because it seemed so penalizing to her to keep eating this way without the needle on the scale even budging.

I suspended the diet for three weeks, because I wanted her to realize that she had the ability to maintain her weight loss. For three weeks she ate differently, for example she added in pizza, and every so often she allowed herself a piece of cake or ice-cream, and much to her delight and surprise she saw that even by herself she had managed to not gain any weight. She had learned how to eat. This realization helped her get rid of her fear of regaining the weight she had lost with so much sacrifice, and she began her diet again feeling much more motivated.

For one week I prescribed her a 1500-Calorie, high-protein and high-lipid diet. In order for foods that contain protein to be digested, a greater amount of energy is required, therefore more Calories are burned up. This diet, if followed for a brief period, gives a boost to the metabolism. I eliminated cereals, pasta and bread. She ate protein-rich foods and as many raw and cooked vegetables as she liked. Moreover, to avoid the formation of ketonic bodies, she also had to have 100 gr of sugar in her diet, so I recommended plenty of fruit.

Her began to lose weight again. She then went back on her 1200-Calorie diet for two months, with two-day intervals every fifteen days of a high-protein diet and one day without dieting. In the final months I introduced a 900-Calorie diet with a two-day break every week.

Caption pg. 102

1500-Calorie diet
pg. 169-73
900-Calorie diet
pg. 157-59

Internal therapy

The first months of therapy was based on dry plant extracts. For her convenience, I chose to prescribe her the plants as a personalized *concoction*.

To stimulate the diuresis during the first months; I advised her to drink *green tea* and camedrio. These have the advantage of not lowering the blood pressure when a person is on a diet. There is a greater risk of this in people who have a tendency for low blood pressure when on a restricted diet.

For the lymphatic drainage, I prescribed her, lymphomyosol, a compound of various homeopathic substances.

For her problems with anxiousness and to help her break down the fat in her abdominal area, I advised her luppolo.

To aid digestion and prevent bloating after evening meals, she had to take an *herbal tea with melissa, fennel, cumin* and *angelica.*

For the few days before her period, to foster diuresis, I prescribed her a *decoction of taraxacum roots, Bermuda grass* and *chicory.*

External therapy

After she had lost ten kilos, I began to apply specific therapy in her abdominal and thigh areas. Although she was losing weight, these areas tended to remain unproportionate and there was no sign of a waistline. I gave her injections of *mesotherapy* using drugs that accelerated the fat-burning process, since the abdominal area was affected more by fat than by cellulite.

Her thighs, especially in the inner thighs, presented cellulite that had accumulated after she had gained weight. I applied five sessions of *ultrasound therapy* and only introduced mesotherapy during the final sessions for the inner thighs, because this area has a greater resistance to eliminating fat.

Caption pg. 89

PHARMACEUTICAL CONCOCTIONS

These are plant substances mixed and prepared by the pharmacist with a medical prescription.
Phvtotherapy
pg. 18493 Mesotherapy
pg. 200-01 Ultrasound therapy

pg. 201-03

In her knees, instead, I applied *mesotherapeutic infiltrations* with substances that increase the resistance of the blood vessel linings (phlebotonic agents) to counteract the tendency for fragile capillaries and followed up on this treatment with *ultrasound therapy.*

Exercise

Isa told me how she decided to be totally committed:

"I had not done any kind of physical activity for 10 years, but ever since you advised me to walk for one hour a day, since this improves circulation, now exercising has become a part of everyday life for me.

I get off the subway one stop early, both on my way to work and when going home.

When I go by the escalator, I take the stairs instead. My lifestyle has changed. I am more active, without overexertion; it is my body itself that asks for more physical exercise, and I've learned to listen to it."

I advised her an exercise workout to do at home to tone up her abdominal muscles and to burn off the fat in that area.

The change

Isa expressed her happiness at the end of the treatment:

"My husband looks at me in a different way.

If I go in a store, I no longer leave with the deep sense of frustration I used to feel. During my lunch break, I don't go to the cafeteria. Instead, I go out shopping for clothes that show off my figure. I'm finally satisfied with my physical appearance. I look at myself in the mirror, which I hadn't done in years, and I don't look the other way to avoid seeing myself, as I used to do. I have change my image. Before, I could only wear pants with an elastic waist and I could have never allowed myself to wear a tight-fitting dress.

One day a co-worker who worked in an office outside of town called me. He had

Caption pg. 90

EXERCISING TO GET INTO SHAPE

The more you exercise the more muscle tissue increases, and fat is burned when the muscles contract. It is the amount of physical exercise one does that determines how many of Calories can be eaten without gaining weight. Exercising is good for the bones, helps eliminate stress, and is also recommended for people who have diabetes. It is, bottom line, a cure-all when practiced in the right amount.

Exercises pg. 194-97

not seen me in years, but he wanted to congratulate me, because he had heard from the others that I had lost weight, looked pretty and was always cheerful. I was amazed and touched, I wasn't used to being at the center of attention."

Isa, with tear-filled eyes as she remembered her past suffering, exclaimed:

"Maybe all these compliments seem like nonsense to you, but for me they represent a fresh burst of energy."

And she continued:

"Now I feel good about myself, I finally like the way I look. If someone does not seem to like the way I dress, it no longer bothers me, what really matters is that now I finally have a positive opinion of myself."

Caption pg. 91

EXCESS WEIGHT
AND SOCIAL PREJUDICE

Excess weight often risks becoming a factor of social prejudice. Our problems can seem enormous and throw us into a downward spiral of despair. We convince our-selves that is is the others who don't accept us, even if a refusal of our own self-image actually starts inside ourselves.
COMPLIMENTS ON YOUR FIGURE
Everybody likes to receive compliments, but especially for those whe are on a diet, they are the tangible proof that all their efforts have been worthwhile. The most appre-ciated compliments, however, are those made by a man to his girlfriend or wife who is dieting to lose weight.

The case of Simona

Simona was a good-looking girl with two lovely blue eyes, but who always had a sad expression on her face. This particular fact, in a girl only 24 years old, struck me as odd; I immediately had the impression she did not feel comfortable with her body.

DIAGNOSIS:

MEDIUM OBESITY, GYNECOID TYPE.

3rd DEGREE COMPACT CELLULITE, located in her thighs and knees. EXCESS WEIGHT: 18.5 kilos.

On her hips and buttocks, she had a problem as a result of localized adipose tissue (localized fat). On the sides and back part of her thighs she had visible cellulite nodules, her knees were overly heavy; in the knee area the cellulite had a pasty texture and tended to show the veined look that is typical of circulatory distress.

From her ankles to her knees she had an edematose type cellulite; the tissue was **full of** liquid and was characterized by a certain pallor and some pain when touched.

Before beginning the treatment, I had her describe her situation to me.

Simona's motivations

I began having weight problems when I was going to junior high school, and between the ages of 13 and 20 I gained 20 kilos. In the last four years I have reached a point where I cannot stand seeing myself this way anymore. I have tried several times to go on a diet, but have always had mediocre results; I would lose a few kilos over a short time, but just as quickly gained them back. To those who tried to convince me to lose weight, I replied angrily that I could have gone on a diet any day, if I had felt like it. This way I only distanced even more the people who were trying to help me.

Another thing that increased the difficulty of my attempts to lose weight was the fact that my base metabolism was so low.

One year ago I made the decision to consult you after an acquaintance of mine described the success she'd had thanks to your anti-cellulite therapies. At the time I weighed twenty-five kilos more than now. With that kind of excess weight, even minimal efforts, such as running to catch a bus or walking up stairs, were a terrible effort for me. Furthermore, I felt awkward around others; often, for example, I avoided getting up to go to the restroom, because I felt everyone would stare at me. In the end I got to the point that I didn't even want to leave the house. With my family I felt fine, because I was surrounded by people who knew me and appreciated me for who I was. The idea of having to be around people who had never seen me, and who might criticize my physical appearance, was unbearable to me.

I selected my friends and tended to associate with people who were fatter than me. The others, I thought, just had to accept me as I was, which, actually, did not happen very often. Only my boyfriend has always appreciated me for who I was—and, naturally, he supports me now in my battle against the extra pounds. My reticence about being around other people bothered him, and he kept trying different ways to play down the problem. He was happy when I told him I wanted to go on a diet, because he wanted me to overcome my complexes.

At home, my father took my weight problem lightly and was decidedly against

---

DEPRESSION AND EXCESS WEIGHT

It is possible for people with excess weight problems to become depressive. They tend to put themselves down and to find situations and associate with people who make them feel comfortable. If they do not find this outside the home, they tend to isolate themselves, sometimes even to the point of not wanting to leave the house anymore. This state of being usually disappears once they draw near to their ideal weight.

It is normal, before making an important decision like that of altering our physical appearance, for us to have to reach a critical point, when we think we can no longer continue this way.

In this case, Simona felt her body had become a bulky obstacle.

Caption pg. 93 Base metabolism

pg. 46

any form of dieting, because he thought that being fat meant being healthy. He couldn't understand how many problems a fat person has to face. My mother, on the other hand, has always encouraged my decision to lose weight, and she was able to understand me because when I gained weight, she did too, perhaps even more so; I went to school, and somehow managed to do even a little physical activity, which her monotonous life as a housewife did not allow her. In the end, despite the criticism from my brother and other relatives who were trying to push me to improve my appearance, I found the strength by myself to get out of this oppressive condition.

Although I was young, I felt old, deprived of the natural energy of a person of my age. I have never worn a mini-skirt and in terms of my looks, have felt very little satisfaction. I decided to go on a diet one day when I was waiting for the mailman to deliver a very important letter for me. The driveway was on a slope and to get to the mailbox I started to run, I was panting, my heart was beating rapidly, I felt I was dying. At that moment I decided to lose weight. It felt as though I had trunks instead of legs. After finding your address, I went down to the subway and dialed your phone number. Even though I was afraid I would be received after a long wait, I managed to set an appointment for the same day. I decided to walk to your

TAKING RESPONSIBILITY FOR ONESELF

When a person who has a problem with excess weight calls the doctor, it means they're aware of their situation and have decided to take responsibility for it.
There will always come a decisive moment in which a weight problem becomes an unbearable burden. The physical problems, but also esthetic factors, lead them to make far-reaching decisions.
If these decisions find their way into our subconscious, and touch our pride, the solution is near at hand. Having people around who are supportive is essential. The greatest love that those near to us can <u>give</u> <u>is to show their trust, encouraging and supporting us when the going</u> <u>gets rough.</u>

Caption pg. 94

DIETING SHOULD BE ENCOURAGED

The main incentive for making important culinary choices is found within the house-hold setting. The members of a person who is trying to lose weight should avoid tempting' them with high-calorie foods, potato chips and sweets. Supporting loved ones in their struggle against excess weight may help them to increase their self-esteem and to continue their diet without feeling deprived. Dietologists, in turn, become an unwelcome coach when they do not talk with their patients enough and do not take their food preferences into consideration.

office, which was a 20 minute walk from my house. After a few minutes, breathless, I promised myself once more that the next time I walked there I would not have to pant anymore, and that's exactly what happened."

The medical treatment

Diet

Simona's weight-loss therapy began with a diet of 1400-1600 Calories per day.

LUNCH I advised her to eat a variety of foods, such as pasta, rice, gnocchi, potatoes, polenta and legumes together with vegetables.

AT DINNER instead, I allowed her to eat meat, fish, cheese and vegetables without having to weigh them. She simply had to keep the dressing, particularly the oil and butter, within the limit of thirty grams per day (three tablespoons).

Initially, she lost about one kilo per week.

After one and a half months, Simona had lost six kilos. After this, I recommended that she sign up at a fitness club because being a student, she led a more sedentary lifestyle, sitting most of the time in university lecture halls and at home.

If she ate at the university, it was difficult to eat the foods indicated in the diet I had suggested, so I advised her to opt, whenever she ate there, for one of the following three menus:

*If she ate at a snack bar grilled sandwich and
fresh-squeezed grapefruit juice OR cappuccino and
a sweet roll.
If she brought her lunch diet soft drink and a sandwich with lean shaved ham OR 500 gr =15 oz of
fruit and 2 yoghurts.*

Caption pg. 95

TASTY AND EASY TO DIGEST

These meals do not make you feel heavy and are easy to digest. University students know that often their classes are back to back without any time for an adequate break. In order to attain good results, it is important to avoid the after-lunch drowsiness that is caused by poor digestion from eating foods that are particularly elaborate, such as lasagne, heavy sauces, fried foods or big meals.

By following her diet, Simona was able to solve the problem of the fat deposits on her hips and buttocks.

Internal therapy

Every month I prescribed her plant preparation

To overcome the nervous hunger that caused her to binge on 'soothing' foods, I prescribed her *California poppy, passiflora* and *valeriana*. In small doses these substances reduce stress, large doses can be used even to treat insomnia. When the right quantities are administered throughout the day, they help attenuate nervous hunger.

To alleviate her morning hypotension (low blood pressure) and to prevent it from worsening while she was on her diet, I prescribed her camedrio and *rosemary*.

For her circulation and cellulite: rusco, betulla and pilosella.

External therapy

As soon as Simona began the anti-cellulite treatment, the shape of her body changed. Before, her thighs were enormous, deformed, now they have slimmed down and Simona can do movements that she was not able to before, such as lifting her legs at right angles or looking at the bottom of her feet with her legs crossed. She has even become more flexible.

After one month of dieting, I started treating her with *ultrasounds* and *mesotherapy*.

The combination of these two techniques is extremely effective in fighting against cellulite. During the first three sessions, 1 proceeded to apply ultrasounds and mesotherapy in sequence. The former had the task of breaking up the tissue affected by cellulitis, the latter of inoculating the medication. The sequential

Caption pg. 96

Photherapy
pg. 184-93
Ultrasound therapy
Ultrasound Therapy pg.201-03
Mesotherapy
pg. 200-01

ultrasounds were applied first on the upper and outer part of the thighs. The upper part of the knees was treated with mesotherapy (injection of lipolytic drugs) and the inner part with ultrasounds.

It is advisable to start the therapy in the knee area or else to treat, in addition to the knees, also the thigh area like I did with Simona. The cellulite in the knees may act as an obstacle to the veins returning the blood from the ankles to the groin.

Exercise

I advise all my patients to walk at least one hour a day and to work out at a fitness club twice a week.

I suggested that Simona do exercises that would work specifically against her cellulite. They can be done for 15 minutes every day or for 30 minutes three times a week.

The change

One of the last times we saw each other, Simona told me how much her mood had improved:

"I am now much calmer, I smile more, I go out, am seen in public, and I enjoy being looked at. Even the way I dress had changed. I no longer want to wear the long and loose clothes I used to put on to hide my body. I stop in front of shop windows with tight-fitting dresses, but I'm still not used to my new size, I still buy clothes that are too big for me.

THE SIZE SAYS IT ALL

When you go down a size this is real and objective proof to confirm even more than the scale that your body size and shape are changing. We should not forget in fact, that for those who are affected by cellulite losing weight can sometimes have a detrimental effect on their figure, since a diet, as drastic as it may be, never completely eliminates the cellulite deposits.

Caption pg. 97

Exercises pg. 194-97

My friends admire me. The sacrifices I make become obvious first of all to myself if others realize the efforts I've made.

There are many temptations, because at the university my friends eat fattening foods that don't go well with my diet, but I always try to stand firm. Sometimes, of course, I have my crises, but in spite of everything I do not let myself give in. I want to show those around me that I am able to resist the temptation, and this gives me enormous satisfaction. I am amazed that I'm not as hungry as I used to be, I eat less than my diet calls for without too much difficulty. I do not feel those nervous cravings I once had and which pushed me to always have something to eat even though I wasn't hungry."

DON'T GIVE IN TO TEMPTATIONS
When you are really motivated, others can tempt you with hundreds of delicacies, but they will not succeed in deterring you from your goal. The admi-

ration of those around you will make you even more determined to follow through. Surround yourself with positive people. If you're on a diet and are afraid you won't be able to stick to it, you need to avoid all situations that will tempt you.

Simona managed to overcome a critical moment during the first days of her diet when eliminating sweets could have created problems. You need to go through a habit-breaking period, just like somebody who wants to quit smoking. After this everything becomes easier. It triggers an awareness that being able to wear a straight skirt without looking fat is no longer a mirage, so even the most appetizing food becomes poison. Try to visualize yourself wearing a sexy dress or in a bathing suit, and imagine how every extra bite will fatten those critical areas and every bite less will mean reaching your objective sooner.

After the first two weeks of dieting, the stomach also gets used to holding less food, and it becomes smaller. This is why, after some time has gone by, the less you eat the less hungry you will feel.

In any case, we must understand the difference between hunger and appetite. Often, those who say 'I'm hungry' are really just in the mood for a certain food. Generally, women feel the urge for sweets, while men tend to prefer salty foods.

Hunger is the need to be nourished. Appetite is the desire to eat certain foods.

At the end of the dietary therapy Simona finally learned to eat a correct and well-balanced diet and to no longer see herself as someone inevitably destined to be a 'fat lady'.

The case of Ferri

The case of this woman, age 57, describes the psychological experience of many people who have gone on diets on numerous occasions with the help not only of dietologists but also of analysts.

Many will be able to relate with her and understand better their love-hate relationship with food, which they always eat in exaggerated amounts.

I will highlight the conflict that arises when someone wants to go on a diet and faces the difficulty of having to maintain the results obtained. Often the consequence of this conflict is a strong feeling of frustration and lowered self-esteem.

Eating correctly must become a way of life.

DIAGNOSIS:

MEDIUM OBESITY, ANDROID TYPE. COMPACT ABDOMINAL CELLLULITE. EXCESS WEIGHT: 20 kilos=44,09 pounds. IRRITABLE COLON.

Adipose tissue in the abdominal area, which had been transformed into cellulite. Inadequate results with weight loss achieved from following a diet. Need to apply localized therapy.

Ferri began to tell her story, in many ways unique.

Ferri's motivations

"I came to you because I needed someone to help me follow a diet by watching over me each step of the way. I had, and still have at times, a difficult relationship with food, a sort of long love-hate affair. I'm over fifty years old and do not like myself much. I would like to be completely different from who I am, and not only on the outside. I need love to live, just as much as the sun, air, light, oxygen and everything else nature offers us to keep us alive. Of course, if I were younger my story would be much simpler, more connected to today's reality; in my case instead, it may seem outdated, might have little meaning for young women of today and the facts may appear twisted, even though it is totally impressed in memory, as real as ever before. I would like to tell you about my childhood, because I'm convinced that was when my preferences came about."

I urged her to continue her story:

"Born one year before the Second World War broke out, in a happy but not very well-to-do family, there was no lack of sickness and hardship. When I was a few months old, I came down with diphtheria and gastroenteritis. According to the mentality of the time, perhaps because during the war there was little to eat, and even ordinary foods like bread, sugar and butter were scarce, a child had to be fat to be healthy. I read recently that the Americans have demonstrated that weight problems arise during childhood, and that the tendency to be overweight continues in adults who as children had excess kilos. I am the living proof of this theory. As a teenager, during the war, my parents sent me to the countryside, near Mantova, to my grandmother whom I loved and who adored me, in a family of only women. I was supposed to stay there only until the end of the war, but life decided differently for us. My father, who had lost his job, was forced to leave Milan with my mother and move out to the country. I lived my adolescence surrounded by much love, like in those fairytales where the protagonists are poor but happy. My childhood memories are all closely connected to food and its good smells.

In the enormous kitchen (as big as a one-room flat today in the city), there was a wooden stove and the water tank, and large windows where I would sit and admire what a wonderful cook my mom was. We had to renounce a lot of things, even foods, during that time, but what mattered most was the quality of the few things we had. There were foods I didn't even know existed, others I had only seen in some shops in town or in other houses. I have often reflected on this love of mine for cooking handed down to me from my family. All my troubles begin here, from the unsatisfied desires back then, the things I wanted but never had. My predilection for sweets, for the smell of food cooking, for the scent that filled my nostrils whenever I entered a greengrocer's shop, the smell of roasted chestnuts in the winter and of tangerines every year on Saint Lucia's' Day, all go back to those days.

Meat was rarely served at our house, and never any red meat. A little more often we could afford polenta and pancakes made only with flour, water and salt, and sprinkled with a bit of sugar, and frugal serv-ings of vegetables, eggs and milk.

Only at Christmas, once the war had been over for several years, did we allow ourselves some little cakes and pumpkin ravioli.

Pudding, creams, pastries and chocolate were only names for me, and the total non-existence of these foods during my childhood, and which children love so much, I believe is the origin of my sweet tooth today.

At that time no one had ever heard of having problems with excess weight or stretch marks, so I was very amazed when during my gym hour in school I saw those ugly lines for the first time on my legs but not on those of my classmates. For parents in those days, the main problem consisted in managing to survive in the most dignified way possible, and in finding enough food to feed their children twice a day.

Now I know that a diet composed only of potatoes, bead and cheese, due to its low nutritional value, can cause debilitation and malnutrition. In fact, I fainted often, in church because of the smell of the candles, and in drugstores from inhaling the odors of medicines used in those days.

After I turned 18 or 21, I began reading articles on nutrition and at the same time to collect cookbooks.

Thus began my yo-yo phase.

The lowest I ever weighed was 45 kilos.

Caption pg. 101

MEMORIES

Memories of food remain more impressed when there is a period of shortage.

From ages 18 to 24, after my first marriage, my weight wavered between 47=103,6 pounds and 49 kilos=108. 1963 was a year when hardships were alternated with better times. Earlier on. I had voluntarily had an abortion, but now I really wanted a child even if for me financially it was not feasible.

My weight kept yo-yoing up and down, even though only slightly, then I got pregnant. My husband was very absent, even emotionally, and I found myself alone having to struggle to overcome the nausea, so I could keep working and not take any medicine.

Those were the years of the terrible Thalidomide. I have always listened to medical advice and have never had problems with taking medicine, but that was the only time in my life when I refused any sort of pills, whether vitamins, products for nausea, or painkillers. It was then that my sciatic nerve began to torment me, and continued to do so even long after the delivery. For the nausea, I decided to eat dry foods: crackers, cookies, bread, which I ate every time the pain became unbearable. During my pregnancy, I gained 22 kilos. After I had the baby, I lost 15 and the remaining 7 over the following months."

She lowered her head, as if to put together her memories, then continued speaking:

"Between 1965 and 1970, after the birth of my son, I never weighed more than 50 kilos.

In 1971, I left my husband. I found a job, but very soon I realized I was not able to handle my new situation without problems. I hid from everyone—or at least tried to—how lonely I was. I worked, did my best as a part-time mother, bearing the burden of my mother-in-law's hatred and that of the rest of my ex-husband's family. I cried and could not even talk to a doctor. I was addicted to sweets. I felt an almost spasmodic craving for them, and my attempts to go against these urges were useless. I began to enter into the tunnel of despair and nervous exhaustion, which became an real, but unwelcome, part of my life. My weight ranged between 53-55 kilos. I felt fat and deformed, so in 1972, for the first time in my life, I sought the help of a dietologist. For a few years I managed to lose weight without much difficulty, and, aware of this, sometimes I whet on total binges, gulping down cream filled cake, carnival pastries and other fattening specialties.

In 1975, I had to be operated for a fibroma in my uterus and ovary. I felt like a dry branch, lifeless, even though I was only 36. Then came a period of good and bad times, not only in my weight, but also in my private and professional life. Perhaps my absolute and unquenchable need for love made me too dependent on the affection of others, so that I was often left helpless.

In 1980, the only remaining ovary stopped working. I went into the 'worst' menopause, which involved terrible headaches, heat flashes that left me soaking wet, mood swings and greater irritability. I felt terrible and comforted myself by eating. This is how my weight began to increase systematically.

Between 1980 and 1983, my second husband began having serious health problems, and after five years of marriage a sudden illness took him away from me in two short months.

I found myself 6 kilos underweight. I began a horrendous phase. My husband and I had been very happy together, and I felt betrayed by him; I had always been the 'sick' one in the family, so I was sure I would be the first one to go. I took his loss as if he had deliberately abandoned me, breaching our agreement. My analyst explained to me that this kind of reaction in similar situations is not uncommon, even though I still don't think I have accepted the idea of his death."

She paused for a moment, overcome by her emotions, then continued:

"Added to this time of bereavement was the difficulty of being a part-time mother, and a series of problems connected to my job, which was not at all suited to me but which I was forced to keep to survive. All in all, I consider myself fortunate not to have fallen into the trip of drug addiction or alcoholism, and to have managed to keep going for the love of my son, thus pushing away the temptation to end my life once and for all.

My drug, so to speak, was food, with which I had built a conflictual love-hate relationship, linked at an emotional level to the ups and downs of life. There were times when small amounts of food were just not enough. My compulsive behavior at the table, which doctors have analyzed on several occasions, came from the sense of emptiness in my stomach that made me unable to stop stuffing myself until I was full.

It was as if it were happening to someone else. It was beyond my control and my common sense. What I felt inside was so intense that at the time my weight meant nothing to me. I tended, nonetheless, to make light of these food binges, which occurred about two times a month, because I was convinced that I could offset them by going on a diet the following day."

FOOD BINGES AND THEIR PSYCHOLOGY

If these binges occur more than three times a week, accompanied by a deep sense of guilt, and at times by self-induced vomiting and the use of diuretics and laxatives, it is necessary to analyze the psychological aspects of these episodes, and possibly resort to the use of antidepressants.

The medical treatment

Diet

The first time we met Ferri told me about her numerous visits to various dietologists and the psychological therapy she had undergone for years. She was very concerned about her periodical binging, which took an enormous effort for her to avoid.

It was at this point that we retraced together her eating habits. Ever since she had started taking an antidepressant, her episodes of exaggerated feelings of hunger (bulimia) had been reduced to once a week. She therefore wanted to know the exact amount of food she should eat daily and to resolve some symptoms that had arisen as a result of bad eating habits. In fact, in addition to her underlying depression, nervousness and frequent insomnia, she was forced to eliminate certain foods as a result of various problems linked to the digestive process.

Milk, yoghurt and cooked green vegetables caused her problems, stimulating bowel movements, whereas bread, pasta, peas and corn caused her frequent meteorism.

There were foods Ferri was not able do without, such as bread-sticks, crackers, bread, cheese, ice-cream and popsicles, while she had for long disliked white and red meats, and neither time nor dieting had changed this.

I reminded her that her meteorism, abdominal pain and alternating periods of constipation and diarrhea were caused by an irritable colon, which she had been diagnosed with ten years earlier.

For the first two months of treatment I prescribed her a diet with no high-fiber foods because of the problems mentioned above. The alternating periods of constipation and diarrhea were frequent, so when she experienced dysentery she had to eliminate raw vegetables and certain kinds of fruit from her diet, and vice versa, introduce more fiber when the acute phase had passed.

The third month of her diet coincided with Christmas, a time of uncontrolled binging according to Ferri. I realized my patient tended to become demoralized often, dramatizing the least little slip in her diet, even if, in fact, she had learned to control her appetite better.

It was on this occasion that, for the first time, the medication she was taking failed in their intent, and the parties, the dinners at restaurants, the holidays, the increase in her daily Calorie intake and the impossibility of reducing that amount in the diet for the following day, made her become totally negative.

In one month she lost only one kilo. For me, it was important that she didn't gain weight, given her history of eating a lot of sweets, especially at a time like Christmas when it is easier to prepare feasts of high-calorie foods. Consequently, in January, I prescribed a computerized diet with a lower calorie intake, 1000 Calories, for her to follow for four days a week. In two months she reached her ideal weight.

I set our next appointment for six months from then. This relieved her, because she was aware of the possibility of a relapse. The maximum amount of weight she was allowed to gain was set at three kilos.

Six months later Ferri came back and told me that maintaining her weight had become a virtual obsession for her, aware as she was of her limits. We had established a trust relationship between us. She ended her diet in March, and in six months she gained three kilos.

The dieting diary she kept showed 1700 Calories for one week, but on weekends her calorie intake went up to 3000-3500.

I prescribed her a 1200-Calorie diet for a week; for her colitis which had worsened, she had to eat potatoes and rice every day until the symptoms disappeared.

For her maintenance period, she followed a 900-calorie diet two days a week, for two months. In this way she returned to her ideal weight.

Internal therapy

For her problems with bulimia and depression, I confirmed the therapy prescribed by her psycho-analyst: the antidepressant *Fluoxetine*.

For the abdominal belatedness and colitis, I prescribed her milk *enzymes, lemon balm, mint* and *orange blossom*.

For her fragile capillaries and continuous infections of the gums, I gave her *rosa caning*.

To combat stress, I recomended her *beer yeast* rich in B *complex vitamins*.

Caption pg. 106

1200-Calorie diet pg. 160-63 900-Calorie diet pg. 157-59
Phytotherapy pg. 184-93

For her dry skin, with a tendency to be atonic, I prescribed her wheat germ oil.

During the final month of dieting therapy I gave her a multi-mineral supplement to take in the morning.

External therapy

When Ferri went down to 70 kilos, I noticed that the circumference of her arms was not getting any slimmer and that her waistline had remained unchanged. For this reason I applied 7 sessions of mesotherapy on a weekly basis in the upper-side and lower abdominal area, so as to stimulate the fatty tissue that had reorganized in part as cellulite.

At home the patient had to commit herself to doing 5 minutes of specific exercises to tone up the area with a special stimulator she purchased at the drugstore. Its function is to transmit an electric impulse to the muscle by means of electrodes.

Exercise

I noticed that over the course of her life Ferri had never mentioned doing any type of sports, or other physical exercise useful for both weight control and better physical health. I, therefore, was very happy when my patient convinced herself that, for her own good, some exercising was essential.

To fight against her lack of muscle tone, I told her to walk for at least half an hour a day.

The stimulator would work to ensure that the tissue was effectively toned up.

The change

At the end of the treatment Ferri told me, not without a pinch of irony, what results she had obtained:

Caption pg.107

Mesotherapy pg. 200-01 _Electric stimulator_ pg. 206

"I have returned to my ideal weight without becoming feeble, but I'm afraid my figure and my willpower do not want to collaborate in the least. Around 10 p.m., at the latest, my stomach no longer listens to reason. I try to keep it under control but it always gets the better of me. I still feel like disaster, I'm better off not thinking about it."

Having said this, she looked at me to see my reaction, and seeing my disappointment, she exclaimed:

"No, doctor, I was only kidding! I now feel like a lion."

"We'll see each other six months from now", I told her. I knew that if she gained weight again, it would not be the fault of bulimia, but of a new life, in which a new love had entered the picture. They are a couple that get along great together and often go out to eat. We tend to eat more when we're not alone.

The case of Raffi

Raffi was a married woman, age 39, with an eleven-year-old son. She came to my office describing her case as one without a solution.

DIAGNOSIS:

MEDIUM OBESITY, GYNECOID TYPE.

CELLLULITE, 4th STAGE, located on the sides and upper back part of the thighs.

EXCESS WEIGHT: 24 kilos=52,91. SAGGING SKIN in both thighs. HYPOTENSION (low blood pressure).

This patient had a problem with excess weight, cellulite and sagging skin on her inner thighs. The cellulite, in its fourth stage, was flaccid and had arisen as a result of dieting begun at age fifteen.

The cellulite in the fourth stage affected the entire thigh and was even more pronounced in her knees. Her calves and ankles were slightly swollen as a result of water retention (edema). Over all, her legs were shapeless and looked like tubes.

Below, Raffi remember the yo-yoing of her weight and the reasons that led her to come to my office.

Raffi's motivations

"When I got married I weighed 64 kilos=141 pounds, after the pregnancy and breastfeeding my baby, I weighed 78=172 poundsl. Then I went up to 90 kilos. Unfortunately, my looks made me feel like a freak of nature. Attempts to go on diets were not lacking in my agenda. Before meeting you, I had started various diets, which had never shown any results, and the more frustrated I felt in my efforts, the more I was bent on eating. I reached my maximum weight two years ago when my mother found out she had a tumor, and together with my brothers I took care of her at home and at the hospital. The loneliness I felt there led me to build a strong 'friendship' with the snack machine, that kept me company especially at night with its coffee and sweet rolls.

I took 'placebo' action to make myself believe I was improving my looks. I bought exercise outfits and slimming creams, but I didn't lose even a bit of weight. I would make incredible sacrifices when forcing myself on a diet of, for example, only milk and yoghurt three times a week, then I would end the diet. I was always hungry and gulped down food like a bottomless pit. Other days I would skip lunch, but then at dinner I'd eat twice as much.

My mother was a good cook. When I went to see her, she always prepared me fancy dishes, but one day even she told me I had gained too much weight and needed to do something about it.

> *HELP OVERWEIGHT PEOPLE WITH TACT*
> *Often loved ones will empathize with the difficulty an overweight person is going through, but do not dare interfere until the problem has reached a critical stage. While it is advisable to avoid forcing a person in this situation with an overly drastic attitude, nonetheless, bringing up the subject of going to see a specialist may help them break out of that vicious circle of helplessness and frustration in which they've become trapped.*

After her death I remembered her words, and 1 decided that I needed to do something that would really work and not stupidly follow the diets found in magazines, or purchase all kinds of slimming creams and girdles, because I had already thrown away a lot of money and had never seen any remarkable results.

I knew that a co-worker of mine was coming to you to lose weight, so I asked her for information. From her enthusiasm I gathered that perhaps I'd finally found what I needed."

She paused, as if to reflect on her past, and then continued:

"I realize that in addition to not being at peace with myself, and not liking how I looked, I didn't even relate well to those around me. I had the impression I was different from other women and I was able to confirm this feeling personally in my relationships with men; my external appearance, it is useless to deny it, has always mattered a lot to me. Even if it was not compliments that I really needed, as nice as these are, but simply to be considered a human being and not a circus animal to point at or ridicule.

My husband had never criticized me openly, but he tried to urge me to exercise and to eat in a well-balanced manner. At the end of a work day, in fact, I would shut myself up at home and eat. If I passed in front of a shop window with my husband and pointed to an outfit that I particularly liked, I understood immediately from his tone of voice that he didn't think it would fit me. At home, I looked at my body in the mirror and just couldn't accept it was mine, I felt depersonalized."

The medical treatment

Diet

Raffi did not eat correctly. In particular, she was not getting her daily requirement of protein per kilo needed to nourish the muscles properly, and this was the cause of her loss of skin tone.

My patient loved to eat, and lack of appetite in her was a sign of sickness. She ate large quantities of high-calorie food, such as potato chips, peanuts, biscuits, and all kinds of snacks. While she was cooking, she would eat 2-3 rolls with the sauce and after dinner would secretly eat more.

She lost weight gradually, 3 kilos a month, compared to 4 or 5 kilos in those who are not affected by flaccid skin.

Initially, she went on a 1500-Calorie diet, so as to lose 600-700 grams per week.

Her daily protein intake was about 90 grams=3 oz.

For years, she had been eating lunch at snack bars or at the cafeteria. Because of her unbalanced nutrition, she suffered from abdominal colics, presumably

Caption pg. 111

IT IS IMPORTANT TO LOOK GOOD

Doing something to improve our appearance helps us feel more secure, because we feel good about who we are.

1500-Calorie diet
pg. 169-73

due to excessive fermentation in the intestines, which causes air to form (meteorism) and is felt after meals.

I established a computerized diet that took into consideration not only her protein requirements, but also the foods that could help her feel better. I gave her general instructions, therefore, on how to reduce the meteorism.

AT THE CAFETTERIA she could eat meat cooked medium to rare, or grilled, but not

boiled (since this is well cooked). She had to eliminate all sauces and eggs, she was allowed cheese only twice a week because, since it is high in salt, it can cause water retention. She could also eat fish baked in aluminum foil.

For the first two weeks, she could have meat with cooked vegetables, no bread, while I advised her not to eat any kind of dessert, fruit and perhaps pudding.

IN THE EVENING, while she cooked dinner, she had hunger attacks, and even when her hunger diminished she felt an incredible urge to devour whatever she could find.

I advised her to eat raw vegetables, which she had to have already washed and chopped for emergencies, or a sandwich made of 60 grams of soy bread and a thin slice of ham.

Internal therapy

Her blood pressure tended to be low, 100/80, whereas most obese people usually have hypertension (high blood pressure). Since she had to lose quite a lot of weight, I had to watch out for her blood pressure, so as not to aggravate my patient's asthenic condition.

To prevent her blood pressure from dropping any lower as a result of dieting, I prescribed her *ginseng* and rosemary.

To improve her digestion and prevent the colics caused by excessive fermentation, I advised her to take *lemon balm, angelica* and *fennel*.

For her anxiousness, *passionflower.*

Caption pg. 112 THINGS To AVOID

Talking while eating,
eating too fast and drinking bubbly water are the main culprits of poor digestion.

Phitotherapy
pg. 184-93

For the water retention, ortosifon.

To help her feel full, *glucomannano*.

To aid her blood circulation, *witch hazel* and *butcher's broom (Ruscus aculeatus)*.

Raffi's skin on her face and body tended to be dry and lackluster, even though she used many moisturizing creams. She had never taken a vitamin complex, so I advised her to take vitamins A and E for one month.

Moreover, she only ate refined foods. B complex vitamins do not fare well when food is processed, since when the bran is removed from rice, wheat, spelt and other gains, the vitamins and minerals are destroyed too; therefore, 1 recommended her a multi-vitamin with B complex vitamins.

I prescribed her bioflavonoid (vitamin P) and vitamin C for her fragile capillaries.

Raffi ate little fruit and vegetables, so she was not getting her daily-recommended amounts of vitamins and minerals.

External therapy

For her flaccid type cellulite, I advised her to apply an anti-cellulite cream every day, in the evening, on the affected area. There are many kinds available on the market, but the best ones are those containing horse chestnut, butcher's broom, escina and caffeine.

I took a picture of the initial situation, in order to better illustrate the program I intended to follow. I examined with her the problem areas to eliminate. Raffi did not even seem to recognize herself in the picture.

After the first month of dieting, I had her begin the external therapy on the affected areas of her legs. In the outer top part of her thighs the presence of capillaries made it essential to begin *mesotherapy* with solutions to protect her blood vessels. At the same time, the inner part of her thighs were treated with *magnetic therapy* for 15 minutes and mesotherapy with *placenta,* combined with weekly intervals of *ultrasounds* and mesotherapy with injections in the folds of her skin. These sequences were necessary to prevent the skin from sagging even more.

After this, I focused my attention on the knee area, starting out with *mesotherapy* and then *ultrasounds* of three Mega Hertz. These heightened the effect of the solutions I injected, and they also enabled the fat trapped in the fibrous tissue to be dissolved, which respond less quickly to the injections otherwise. I wanted to reduce the circumference of her knees even more so they would not have that tube shape.

After 8 enhanced sessions, in which I always prolonged the therapy sessions themselves, we began to see the first results, especially in her knees. Naturally, the patient continued to follow her diet throughout the therapy.

I the following sessions I applied *magnetic therapy* to her knees as well. This brought about an increase in the local circulation, useful for draining excess liquids, in addition to micro-massaging the muscles and enhancing skin trophism.

In the final sessions I applied *electro-toning therapy,* which causes the muscles to contract by means of a device that reproduces the nervous stimulation of the muscle, which causes the muscle to move and tone up the area. After this, I added local injections with *placenta* along the inner thighs.

Exercise

After two months of therapy, I advised Raffi to purchase a special device to do exercises at home that would make her thighs firmer. Every day she had to work

Caption pg, 114

Mesotherapy. 200-01 Magnetic therapy pg. 205-06 Ultrasounds
pg. 201-03
Electro-toning therapy
pg. 206

Inner thigh firmer
pg. 197

out for five minutes, any time of the day, even while watching TV. After one month, we started seeing the first results.

After she had lost 15 kilos, I suggested she sign up for an aerobics class. She had never done any sports, so she had to start up gradually, 20 minutes at a time until she could work out for one hour. Her desire to improve her looks compelled her to exercise regularly and to go to the fitness club three times a week. When she went back home, she wasn't hungry.

The change

At the end of her therapy, Raffi beaming announced:

"Consulting your clinic has done wonders for me. I have learned how to eat and to prepare meals for dinner guests with non-diet foods without feeling tempted by them. Even my husband is convinced. It happened in a strange way. He saw me in front of a tray of sweets and noticed that I didn't eat any because I didn't feel the need. He couldn't help expressing words of sympathy for me, but I readily told him that even though I had been foolish before, I was now determined to contain myself. I no longer eat out of habit. I only eat the first or the second course, and I always drink plenty of water.

I understood that my body was changing for the better and the first confirmation of this was at work. I began to notice co-workers looking at me with interest. Now, as I turn 40, I have men courting me, one of whom, a very handsome man, even told me outright he wanted to have an affair with me. I joke about this with my husband, I like to tease him and make him a bit jealous. Now I enjoy wearing sexy lingerie and I take better care of my body. My marriage has always been happy, but today I'm absolutely sure my change has strengthened it, even if, as my husband says, looks are not the only thing that matter in a woman. I know I have given him something extra. My husband has always played soccer, worked out at gyms, gone to the swimming pool whenever possible, and he is a really

Caption pg. 115

AEROBICS

This type of exercise requires the body to use a large amount of oxygen and enhances the capacity of the cardiovascular system.

THE GOLDEN RULE

Often, when on a diet, people are not able to eat the quantities of food on their daily chart. That is why it is better to eat the first course and the raw vegetables or a large serving of grilled fish and vegetables.

good-looking forty-year-old. Finally, he comes with me to stores, gives me advice while I try on clothes and sometimes he surprises me, buying me modern or chic little outfits. This summer I even wore transparent lacy tops and wrap-around skirts. I felt glamorous.

This change in my physical appearance has been followed by changes in my daily life too. Being happy for me means being able to walk by my husband's side without thinking I make him ashamed. Some people have even turned around to look at me, which hadn't happened to me in a long time.

Some friends I hadn't seen in years told me I smile more now and am less unsociable, and they even find me younger looking.

All of this makes me happy and angry at the same time, because I realize what a huge gap exists between how differently people consider me compared to before. I cannot help thinking how empty and unhappy life seemed when I was overweight.

In June, I went to the seaside for a week and finally, after such a long time, I was not ashamed to wear a bathing suit and sunbathe in public, after so many years of living as a hermit.

Raffi was visibly satisfied with her success. In fact, she continued:

"I am glad I sent several of my colleagues to you, since they, like me, felt very comfortable with you. Since you let your patients talk, you are able to understand their problems and try each time to provide interesting ideas so that dieting doesn't become a bore or a burden but rather as a correct way of eating, which even people who don't have weight problems should abide by. Before, when I walked around, only skinny people caught my eye. Nowadays, instead, I notice that there were many girls with excess kilos. I would like to stop them and tell them my story and convince them to deal with the problem while they're still young.

I can imagine what they're going through, I was the same way."

On Raffi's last day of therapy she looked a bit sad; I couldn't understand, so I asked her why. She answered:

"You see, doctor, you were not only a good doctor for me but also a real friend, who helped me find myself again."

The case of Patrizia

Patrizia entered through the doorway of my office with a decidedly depressed expression on her face and the look of someone who has nothing to lose if she leaves this life. She walked slowly, with a hesitant and awkward gait, hindered by large-sized clothes that made her look even heavier.

DIAGNOSIS: MEDIUM OBESITY. CELLLULITE, 4th STAGE, located on her hips and the upper part of her thighs. EXCESS WEIGHT: 29 kilos=63,9 SIDEROPENIC ANEMIA (iron deficiency).

The cellulite was in its fourth stage. The nodules were large and painful to the touch, located on the hips, on the outer and back part of the thighs.

Her story illustrated the situation, especially the psychological situation, she was in.

Patrizia's motivations

"I feel like a ball whose diameter is rounder in the middle, and my hips and thighs seem full of holes like Swiss cheese. These craters on my skin are not only ugly, they also hurt me; I feel a terrible heaviness in my legs and the discomfort is continuous, whether I'm standing still or walking, going from my ankles all the way up to my groin. If I stoop down, my feet turn blue and I start having cramps after a few seconds. This scared me a great deal, because my father was operated for varicose veins and I'm afraid I have a circulatory problem too. I'm terrorized at the thought of having an operation. When I was 18, I was fairly thin, weighing 52 kilos 114,6 pounds. I began to gain weight at age 21, when I was expecting my first daughter. During my pregnancy I gained about 22 kilos=48,50 pounds. After my daughter was born, I weighed 80 kilos=176,3pounds, and I began one of many, useless, weight loss diets.

At the outset, it seemed as though everything was fine. I was radiant, because I'd managed to lose 10 kilos=22 pounds, but soon after going off my diet, I gained every last ounce back. I let some time go by and then tried again with some other diets, but without much success. I kept on changing dietologist, but every attempt ended in failure. I weighed around 65 Kilos=143 pounds.

I gave birth to another little girl, and during that pregnancy I tried to watch my weight more carefully. I gained 'only' 14 kilos. It was after my daughter's birth that my situation went from bad to worse. I began to gain weight continuously and I felt as though I were rising like dough. I was a big balloon, and weighed 85 kilos.

So, I decided for the umpteenth time to lose weight and I went to a specialized center where the therapy consisted in wrapping myself up with bandages soaked in a cold substance. They also prescribed me a non-personalized diet that helped me lose seven kilos over a year and a half.

I was always grouchy, nervous, depressed, dissatisfied with life and everything around me. Nothing worked for me, and the more I decided not to eat the more I ate.

WEIGHT LOSS AND PHYSICAL AND PSYCHOLOGICAL HEALTH

A low self-esteem magnifies and exaggerates our problems and causes depression. In such a state of mind it is easy to adopt an anti-social behavior toward loved ones, coworkers and friends. When we lose weight, this attitude ceases, and those around us notice both a physical and a psychological change in us.

In this way, I ended up weighing 82 kilos=180,7 at age 33. I had a morbid attraction to food and ate continuously, out of a nervous habit.

I was angry with the whole world. I felt ashamed of myself and tended to stay away from others. I didn't want to leave the house anymore, not even with family friends. I didn't want my husband to have to be ashamed of his wife. I was disgusted and revolted at myself.

Physically, I was very tired and depressed. It often happened that, before falling asleep, I would nurture negative thoughts that diminished even more my already non-existent self-esteem.

THE SUBCONSCIOUS

There is a part of our unconscious mind called the subconscious. Addressing it with negativity may have disastrous consequences. It appears that success in our daily activities is directly related to the number of positive phrases transmitted to the subconscious during times of quiet and reflection and before falling asleep.

Here is an example to understand how to help oneself if I think I'm not anxious, the subconscious does not receive the not' and understands only I'm anxious'. Positive messages must be sent, such as I am calm', I'm a good person, % look pretty' and I'm capable'.

My husband didn't talk with me much, because he saw me so preoccupied and demoralized.

I thought he didn't care about our relationship anymore. My weight had become an enormous problem; I was convinced there was no way of going back to how I was before. One day, however, a friend of mine told me how she had overcome her weight problem by following your advice and I told myself: 'Why shouldn't I do the same?'

My eating behavior was certainly not normal (compulsive). When I cooked for my family, I wasn't hungry and at dinner would not eat anything, or else only a small portion. Then, after dinner, while watching TV, or while I was ironing, I felt a need for something, perhaps out of boredom or hunger, and I would start to munch on crackers, sweet rolls or bread sticks. The urge to eat was stronger than my willpower and made me overdo it.

My husband tried to convince me to eat fruit, and I would eat dried fruit. I felt a tremendous need to have something solid to chew. 'How fat I am!' I would tell myself and meanwhile open the fridge and eat. I thought, 'I can't help it, and I kept eating. I always felt I was in need of something. The impulsive eating varied from day to day. The thought of going on a diet only made me eat more. The fact that I came to you before the Christmas holidays, a time loaded with temptations, shows me that my suffering was what made me decide. Inside, I repeated to myself that this would be my last attempt. I was a bit scared, but now you've given me courage."

Caption pg. 120

COMPULSIVENESS

In psychology this term is used for a violent impulse, a more or less conscious urge, accompanied often by feelings of anguish, that compels a person to behave in a certain way.

The medical treatment

Diet

I decided to prescribe her a personalized diet that would take her times of weakness for sweets into consideration, so that she wouldn't have the impression she was in a labor camp, thus defeating every attempt as had indeed occurred on her other diets.

I had her give me as much information as possible about her eating habits, the places and times when she had fits of nervous hunger. I then dealt with correcting her way of eating. I prescribed her diet of 1300-1600 Calories, with an extra 300 Calories for when she felt a need for certain foods. This was to prevent the guilty feelings for having eaten more. I did not ask her to analyze her feelings during those 'emergency' times; with time she would learn to avoid them. She could be compelled to eat that 'extra food' out of hunger, boredom or anger.

AT NOON she could follow her diet, even having lunch at the cafeteria at work. Unfortunately, there was little choice of grilled or steamed food. The problem was solved by limiting the amount of fattening foods and opting for meat or fish without sauces or gravy. Fortunately, there was a large choice of vegetables that she liked a lot.

IN THE EVENING she had to weigh her pasta, bread and other carbo-hydrates. Four times a week, always in the evening, she could also have a second course of low-fat cheese or an egg or fish (sole, trout or salmon).

Once a week she could eat pizza.

During her therapy, Patrizia told me how her decision to finally lose weight had been welcomed at home:

My husband and daughters do not follow my diet, but they point out every time I get off track, without at the same time getting me all anxious. I didn't expect so much help from them!

Caption pg. 121

Diets
pg. 157-83

My husband tries to take me to restaurants where I can follow my diet without any trouble."

My patient had some moments of panic when she got down to 75 kilos, because for a few weeks the scale didn't budge. Disappointed, she told me:

"It's happening like the other times. I get to a certain weight and then my body refuses to lose more. And yet, I'm still following the diet. Can you explain this to me?"

Very calmly and confidently, I answered:

"Because You are eating more than what your diet calls for."

Very calmly and confidently, I answered:

"Because you are eating more than what your diet calls for."

WITH YOUR DOCTOR, BE SINCERE

Often people who are dieting are ashamed to admit they ate more than they should have, and prefer to lie. The doctor should not make them feel guilty, but neither should he pretend the patient is right, since this creates a vis-cous circle that causes the therapy to fail.

I left her with this statement until she confessed to me that she had grown weary with the diet and in the evening tended not to follow my advice, allowing herself excess Calories.

This awareness, in addition to accepting the responsibility of being open with her weakness, allowed me to evaluate how much she really to continue the dietary therapy.

In order to help her in this second phase of the diet, I gave her a prescription for tablets containing *dexfenfluramine,* to take with a 1200-Calorie diet this time.

Internal therapy

To revitalize the skin on her skin and body, I prescribed her a multivitamin with *vitamin A, vitamin C, vitamin E, Zinc* and *Selenium.* This compound has an antioxidant effect, i.e. against free radicals, which are responsible fro the aging process and perhaps for the onset of some tumors.

Caption pg. 122

1200-Calorie diet
pg. 160-63

For the constipation, I prescribed her *frangula, mallow* and *ispaghul.*
For her headaches she had to take *escolzia, hawthorn (Crataegus oxyacantha)* and passionflower.
For her meteorism, *fennel, mint* and *milk thistle.*

External therapy

I put her on a therapeutic program to treat her cellulite and problem legs. Already after four sessions we began to see the first results. My patient was happy and decided to continue. She herself told me:

"I lost several kilos feeling good about myself and with others. I did not find it hard to do this therapy once a week. My daughters and my husband, seeing the first results, encouraged me to continue telling me this was the right solution to my problem."

The first eight sessions were focused on the thigh area, the most affected area. The treatment consisted in applying *mesotherapy followed by laser therapy,* focusing the infrared rays on the painful nodules. After the seventh week, the pain had not gone away yet. I then used *ultrasound therapy,* followed by mesotherapy, with solutions to protect the blood vessels, and in the following weeks, products that dissolved fat (lipolytic substances).

The combined therapies worked together, enhancing their effect considerably and therefore speeding up the results. In all, she had 23 combined sessions.

Exercise

I advised Patrizia to walk for at least one hour a day.

she told me she walked half an hour at lunchtime, with other co-workers, and half an hour in the evening when she walked the dog or went out with family members. She discovered with satisfaction that this relaxed her a great deal.

Caption pg. 123

Phytoterapy
pg. 184-93

Mesotherapy pg. 200-01 *Laser therapy* pg. 204-05 *Ultrasound therapy* pg. 201-03

She didn't want to sign up for exercise classes because of her past experience. At a non-medical center, for a year and a half, she had gone through 150 sessions of 'fat dissolving' bandaging and exercised three times a week. Her impression was that her muscles had grown larger and that the cellulite showed even more.

The change

At the end of the therapy, Patrizia described her new situation to me:

"I am 36, and I finally feel good about myself. My life has changed, I'm a new person, and I finally leave the house confidently, without feeling ashamed. I talk with everyone, go out in public without worrying and no longer turn down dinner dates with friends. Even with the people at work I have established a good relationship. They keep on paying me compliments, telling me I look younger. Before this did not happen; it is as if I had not existed until today and suddenly had appeared as a new employee. This makes me feel happy.

Even my problem with eating too much on days when I have nothing to do had disappeared. Since I like being around others, I am no longer tempted to eat between meals. In the evening for me it is more important to talk with my family or go over to a friend's house.

I feel free from all constraints. It's as if I had taken off layer upon layer of fat. Before. I felt 'trapped', almost asphyxiated by all the fat that cushioned my body. actually, my biggest success was to have managed to discuss this problem with my husband and in this way to communicate on a more intimate level with him. When I asked him why he had never said anything about my obesity, and I admitted to him that I was convinced he didn't care about me and that I suffered a lot from his indifference, he answered me: 'I didn't dare say anything, because I was afraid that you would do something rash. I loved you before, but now I love you even more. You've changed for the better, not only physically, but also in your character. If I'm not careful, someone will take you away, as beautiful as you are on the outside and inside'."

Patrizia smiles happily. She tells me she is overjoyed and knows she deserves to feel this way:

"Our marriage relationship has improved, and now there's even a pinch of mischief in me. I admit, I have fun making him die of jealousy. After all, men should always be kept on tenterhooks, right?"

The case of Caterina

Caterina came to my clinic because for the last three years she'd had a problem with her weight and blood pressure (140 maximum and 125 minimum). Her cardiologist had advised her to consult me.

DIAGNOSIS: SERIOUS OBESITY. CELLLULITE, 4th STAGE, located in the lower abdomen and inner thighs. EXCESS WEIGHT: 29 kilos=64 ponds .

GLOBULAR ABDOMEN, lacking skin tone. HYPERTENSION.

On the abdomen, as a result of the increase in adipose tissue, 3rd degree cellulite had also formed on top of the existing fat. The situation was aggravated further still in the lower abdominal area, which was affected by sagging skin.

In the inner thigh area there was cellulite in its fourth stage combined with loss of skin tone.

Caterina's motivations

"I need to lose weight. I have high blood pressure", she began." Physically, I feel huge. I gained a lot of weight after my pregnancy, and due to stress-related problems, I eat without restraint. My tachycardia and heart compression occurs constantly, to the point that one night I had to be rushed to the hospital, where I was told the problems were caused by stress, which my cardiologist then confirmed. Unfortunately, because of this problem, my blood pressure increased, reaching a peak of 220 over 130. My cardiologist treated me, but at the same time sent me to you with the utmost urgency, telling me that the results would only last if I lost weight. I am obese. I even have difficulty breathing. My anxiousness grips me and the tranquillizers make me a total idiot. Plus, my blood pressure has become a nightmare. It goes up every time I get the least bit angry, and deep down there is a lot of anger in me because of my family situation. Food has become my refuge for escaping from the stressful situation at home. In addition to solving my physical problems, I want to return to my ideal weight to get back at my husband.

He is having an affair with another woman, and I 've had to act as if I didn't know, despite my suspicions. But, in the end, I discovered the truth and I framed him. A person gave me the other woman's address, so I was able to catch him in the act. She was ugly, so I couldn't help jeering at him, although I felt humiliated. I am a dynamic woman, and when I'd reached my limit, I exploded. I grabbed my husband by his jacket and hurled him against a wall, saying: 'I was an attractive girl, I could have had many men, but I chose you. Now I'm going to get in shape and show you what I'm capable of'."

Certainly, Caterina, taking such a firm stand, and not becoming a victim, trying to forgive and be forebearing—too often the case of many women—she managed to find the courage to face a situation, whose consequences were unknown, and turn it around in her favor. She was not about to share her husband with his lover and was, on the contrary, ready to face a divorce. This drastic decision scared her spouse considerably.

Diet

It was this same Caterina who expressed to me her fears about weight-loss diets:

"Unfortunately, I have always hesitated to go on a diet, because I enjoy eating well, and in particular, I'm afraid of what it will do to my stomach. It is fat and tends to sag. In the lower abdomen two ugly rolls of fat have formed."

Her initial diet called for 1200 Calories. She had to eat low-salt foods, rich in potassium, which is found in vegetables, and get her protein from fish as opposed to other sources, because it is high in polyunsaturated fats.

Caption pg. 127

1200-Calorie diet
pg. 160-63

After the first month of therapy, my patient was able to lose 5 kilos=11 pounds. Her blood pressure returned to acceptable levels (130185).

After this, the next three kilos were lost gradually to give the skin time to regain elasticity.

Internal therapy

For her blood pressure, the water retention and the palpitations caused by stress, I prescribed *hawthorn*, *Bermuda grass* and *betulla*.

For her abdominal pains induced by poor digestion, I gave her *carbon vegetal* and *lavender*.

External therapy

On a weekly basis, I performed *mesotherapy* with lipolytic solutions on her abdomen.

To solve the problem in her thighs, mesotherapy was applied on the protruding folds of skin and *ultrasounds* used on the inner parts.

In all, 1 did 12 combined sessions.

Exercise

I had her purchase a stimulator at the pharmacy for passive exercise. Its purpose is to cause the muscles to contract. I asked her to use this machine on her abdominal area every day for five minutes, so as to increase the volume of and tone up the muscle tissue.

The change

Her blood pressure stabilized, after a certain period of taking the medication prescribed by her cardiologist, around a maximum of 170 and a minimum of 95.

Caption pg. 128

Phytotherapy
pg. 184-93

Mesotherapy pg. 200-01 Ultrasounds pg. 201-03
Electric stimulator

Her blood pressure tended to vary, rising to previous the levels whenever she had to face stressful situations. The tachycardia and at times the episodes of arrhythmia appeared with increasing frequence at times not directly linked to states of anxiousness, perhaps due to the pressure exerted on her heart by the fat in her abdomen.

After one month of dieting, her blood pressure stabilized around 120 (high) over 80 (low).

The tachycardia disappeared once the patient had lost 10 kilos =22 pounds.

Even in her family the tension and stress diminished little by little.

"My husband has changed; he is no longer ashamed to take me around. He often invites me out to dinner and on his business trips, and he has become more attentive. I no longer feel the need to threaten him", concluded Caterina, laughing with an air of satisfaction and confidence.

The case of Valentina

Valentina was a nice girl, age 24, with a lively personality. Her weight problems developed early, when she was still a little girl.

DIAGNOSIS: SERIOUS OBESITY. CELLLULITE, 4th STAGE, located in the upper part of the thighs. EXCESS WEIGHT: 30 kilos=66 pounds.

The obesity was the gynoid type, with accumulated fat in the lower part of the body, where compact cellulite had formed in the trochanteric area.

The patient let me know how much she was suffering from her excess weight.

Valentina's motivations

"At elementary school and junior high my classmates made fun of me because I was somewhat chubby, but this didn't bother me so much. My mother, on the other hand, was disturbed by my appearance, and continually repeated that 1 was obese so, in order not to hear her grumbling, I started dieting at age fourteen. I remember an ice-cream diet 1 did which made me even fatter than before! I weighed 84 kilos=185 pound. I wore a size 52 for pants, and to buy an outfit I had to go to a specialized shop for maxi-sizes. Thin people can find clothes for every occasion on sale; I, however, was forced to spend much more.

At parties no one asked me to dance, so to be accepted by the others, I had to have a great personality. I was appreciated for my character, which was so spontaneous.

I admired the girls who were pretty and thin, but this did not motivate me to lose weight, because I got along fine with others and always felt at the center of attention.

I only decided to do something when I turned twenty. I knew that when I was old I could develop problems in my bones, just like my grandmother who is obese (you have to sacrifice more to live your old age better!); in addition, I was competing with my friends who were models. I had the clear goal of demonstrating that I too could become as beautiful as they were. That way, I thought, I would look good in my eyes and in my mother's, and she would finally be happy with me. It was during that last diet that I confessed to her how attacked I had felt by her until then, and she was hurt by this. I met my boyfriend when I weighed the most ever. My dearest friends are petty girls, but they told me they would prefer to weigh 20 kilos more, to be accepted for who they really were. It is nice when our worth is not measured only by our looks. My boyfriend did not support me much in my decision to lose weight, he didn't want me to get too thin, because he was afraid of losing me."

The medical treatment

Diet

Valentina did not eat correctly. Usually she made rich sauces for her pasta, used plenty of oil and had a habit of topping her cake with ice-cream, thus increasing considerably the Calories she ate.

She had started going on a diet by herself and had managed to lose a few kilos, but when she realized that the saddlebags did not disappear and her body had lost muscle tone, she had quit her diet and immediately gained weight again. It was at this point that she came to me.

She had suffered for years from stomach aches caused by gastritis, probably as a result of eating smoked meats, for which she had a weakness.

It was not difficult to implement a therapeutic program with Valentina, because already by herself she had learned by heart the calorie content of many foods. I did, however, have to teach her which foods could be eaten together. The first two weeks I eliminated all high-fiber foods from her diet, since these cause abdominal pains as a result of excessive fermentation. When high-fiber foods are eaten, they must be introduced gradually, since the intestines must get used the content of indigestible fiber. Moreover, it is important to drink a lot of water, because this helps the digestive tract become less irritated.

Therefore, during the first two weeks, she had to weigh her food and follow a 1500-Calorie diet.

I also advised her to limit the amount of sugar she ate.

SUGAR

Sugar is an instantly absorbed nutrient. One gram contains 4 Calories.

Often when adding sugar to our drinks, we don't watch the quantity. In general, we consume an average of about ten teaspoons per day. One teaspoon contains roughly 40 Calories, which means can easily consume up to 400 Calories, as much as a medium serving of pasta.

For people on a low-calorie diet it is preferable to use artificial sweeteners. There are various kinds available in stores: saccharine, cyclamate, D-trypto-phan, aspartame, potassium acelsufame and others,

Also, for several years my patient had been suffering from headaches, probably caused by stress or by an excessive use of products containing glutamate (found, for example, in bouillon cubes), which I advised her to use less.

After this, I instructed her to alternate, over a six-month period, a 900-Calorie diet that she was to follow for three weeks, and a 1500-diet for one week. Once a week she could choose a menu of her choice, such as pizza with ham, or an ice-cream for dessert, or chocolate to satisfy her sweet tooth.

Internal therapy

For the constipation, caused by an insufficient amount of exercise and a lack of

Caption pg. 132 **1500-Calorie diet**

pg. 169-73
900-Calorie diet
pg. 157-59

fiber and liquids, I also prescribed her, on top of her diet, an *herbal tea with frangula, fennel,* and *lemon balm.*

She had to take *milk enzymes* for two weeks, at lunch and dinner, to restore the bacteria in her intestines and alleviate the symptoms of poor digestion.

To reduce the belatedness at mealtimes, I had her takes prescription tablets of *pancreatin* and *dextran.*

External therapy

I advised my patient to apply an *anti-cellulite cream* in the morning and evening.

The first three therapeutic sessions involved *mesotherapy* and *laser therapy,* while in the last seven I combined mesotherapy *and ultrasound therapy.*

The first combined technique was used to reduce the *edema* and pain, and to stimulate the blood circulation. The area treated was always the side of the thighs, where she had visible saddlebags.

The combination of mesotherapy and ultrasounds was carried out as follows:

1) mesotherapy with a single needle using the following substances: anesthetic, physiological solution and a lipolytic substance;

2) cellophane wrapped around the area treated with mesotherapy to prevent the gel used to transmit the ultrasounds from coming in contact with the blood from the injection.

3) low-frequency ultrasound therapy for the first five minutes, and higher frequencies in the last fifteen minutes.

When this sequence is utilized—first the mesotherapy and then the ultrasounds, not the other way around—careful attention must be paid to the patient's tolerance level, since this technique may cause some discomfort and lead to the

Caption pg. 133

Phytotherapy
pg. 184-93

Mesotheranv pg. 200-01 *Laser therapy* pg. 20405 *Ultrasound therapy* pg. 201-03

formation of tiny burns a few millimeters long if the frequencies are set too high. The sequential method is the most effective one, since it heightens the effect of the ultrasounds, but demands the constant presence of a doctor and his supervision if the patient shows any intolerance.

Valentina soon realized how effective these medical therapies are:

"The shape of my legs has changed. I have seen how absolutely necessary these therapies are, since I noticed, as put on a pair of pants, a substantial difference in my figure compared to two years ago, when I weighed, like I do now, 65 kilos=143 pounds; this has been possible through the application of localized therapy."

Exercise

After four months of dieting, Valentina signed up at a fitness club, where she worked out 3 times a week for one hour.

The change

Before concluding her last visit, Valentina told me how much her new physical condition had influenced her life positively:

"I'm happy because my headaches disappeared already after the first weeks of dieting, having eliminated the glutamate from my diet. In fact, previously I used little salt, and when I prepared a sauce or a soup I would regularly use bouillon. Moreover, I was a regular customer at chinese restaurants, where these substances are widely used.

I have no longer felt any pain in my bones. The arthrosis, caused by the extra 30 kilos I carried around, has stopped and I, who used to walk like an old lady, have now become as agile and lively as when I was 24.

But for me the greatest satisfaction has been to be able to wear a size 42. It was my desire and I made it, because I lost not only weight, but also several centimeters right around my thighs.

I am even admired for my figure. My father admitted to me only now that before losing weight he thought I looked horrible. My boyfriend loved me before too, but he says the change in me is incredible. Many do not recognize me. I have fun going out, being around people I haven't seen in a while and watching the way they react to seeing me so different.

I like being at the center of attention; after all, my zodiac sign is a Leo!"

Then she asked me: 'What sign are you?' I answered: 'Does it matter?'

I like being at the center of attention after all

Then she asked me; 'What sign are you'? I answered: 'Does it matter?'

'Astrology is a hobby of mine, she admitted, and I'm convinced stars influence our relationship, our jobs and our success that the stars

I burst out laughing 'I'm an Aquarius, and I know it is a sign that looks to the future…happy?

The case of Marinella

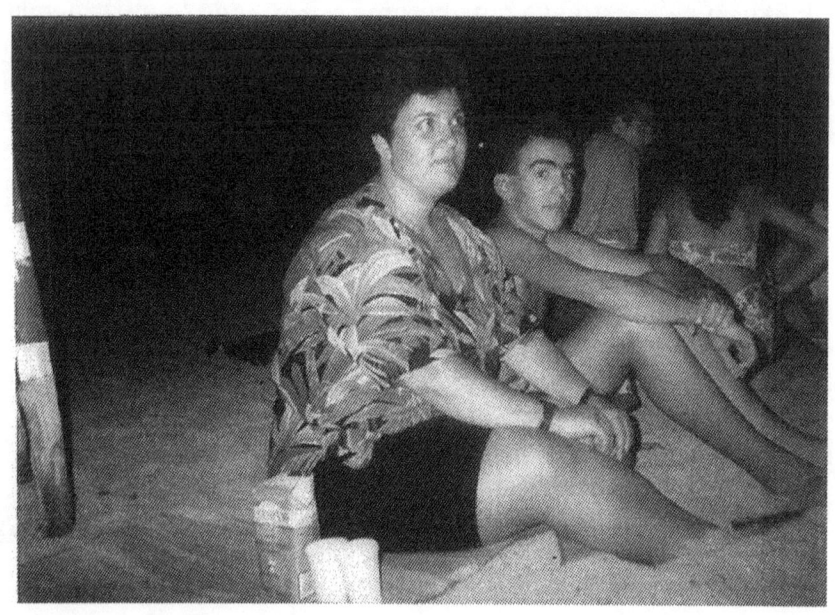

marinella before bw

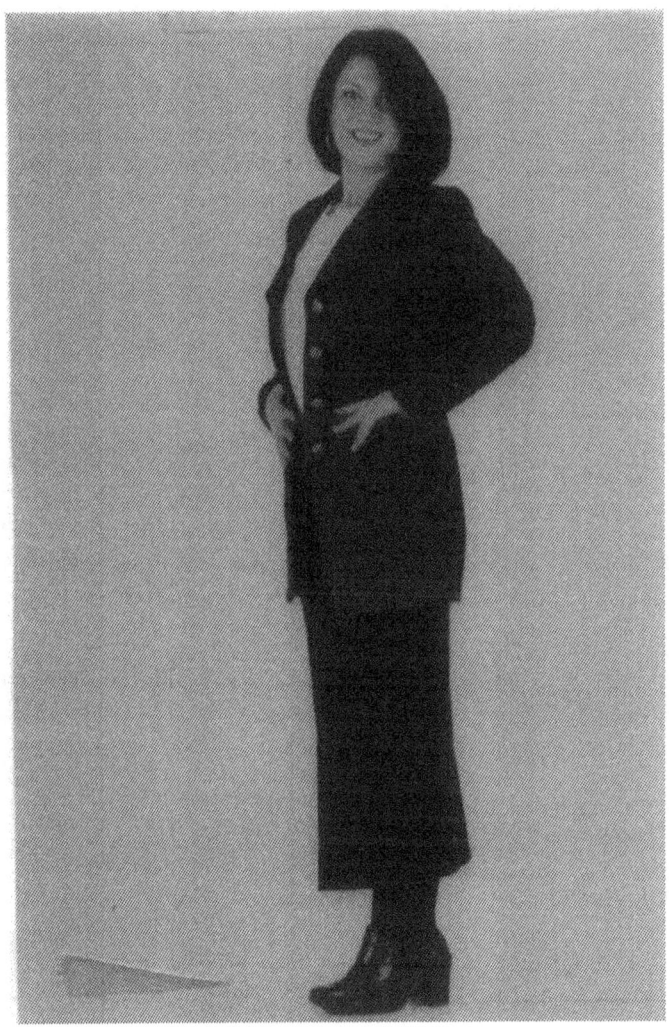

marinella after bw

Marinella was 30 years old and had a bored and sullen look on her face when she came through the door of my clinic. Already after her first visit her face lit up with hope.

DIAGNOSIS: SERIOUS OBESITY. CELLLULITE, 4th STAGE, located on both thighs. EXCESS WEIGHT 50 kilos=110 pounds.

LOSS OF SKIN TONE on both thighs. HIGH CHOLESTEROL.

Marinella's obesity was characterized by an even distribution of body fat. In her thighs there was a mix of cellulite in its fourth stage and fat tissue.

During the course of her therapy, Marinella came to understand better the causes of her physical condition, actively involving herself in the process of changing it.

Marinella's motivations

"Once at three in the morning I found myself devouring a container of icecream, and while I was eating it I looked at myself in the mirror and told myself: 'I can't go on like this'. 1 looked enormous, a shapeless bulk. It was the first time I observed my body, because I never looked at it before. Even in front of a mirror I only saw my face, which I took good care of. Everyone says I have a pretty face, but I wore dark, loose-fitting clothes, almost as if to make my body as unnoticeable as possible, since I rejected it."

HOW WE PERCEIVE OUR BODY

Perceiving our body as something foreign to us only serves to increase our difficulty with integrating well socially, and causes us to be more anxious about our ability to handle situations we think are only suited to thin people, such as wearing a bikini, running or dressing up in a tight outfit. It is not possible to live in the future, but living consciously in the present will allow us over time to achieve what we most desire.

Whenever I walked, I got tired immediately and was short of breath. I was ashamed to show myself in public and was convinced that others looked at me because I was so fat and huge. I didn't want to

go out because I had the impression people only considered my physical appearance.

Passing in front of shop windows, I glanced in that direction but
never stopped to look, because I was afraid people would think: 'What
is she doing looking at things that don't fit her?' At age 25, I wore a
size 60. Being that heavy at this age meant I could only wear wide
skirts that made me look even fatter, but that was the only thing that fit
me. Since age 15, I have always weighed over 100 kilos, and as a little
girl I was nicknamed 'fat gypsy', because I have dark skin and hair.

When I was around my friends I never spoke up, because I was
ashamed to stand out. Ever since I was a little girl, I have always been at
the center of attention for my huge size, and this made me feel terrible.

I was dominated by everybody; in my job as an assistant cook,
whenever they asked me to taste something, I did it as if it were an
order, and if someone yelled out me I didn't react. I just opened the
fridge and took out my anger eating.

I understood this was wrong and I blamed others. I thought I could
punish those who made me suffer by showing them it was their fault if
I ate, and this happened even if I wasn't hungry. Once, for example, I
knew that there was a jar of Nutella (chocolate-hazelnut spread) in the
cupboard, and even though I had just finished eating, I couldn't stop
thinking about it. I promised myself I would have a taste before going
to bed, and instead I devoured half a jar. On other occasions, I would
buy a container of ice-cream and gobble it down greedily in a matter of
minutes. Often I would get up during the night with the urge to snack
even though I wasn't hungry, and if I didn't find what I wanted, I
would even go so far as to cook a plate of pasta.

My sisters would tell me that if I did not lose weight no man would
want me, but I did not react, because I was sure that I would never be
able to reach a normal weight. 1 weighed 117 kilos, and according to
weight/height charts, I was in the category of serious obesity.

My mother was obese too. After her death I went through a period
of apathy. I quit my job and, almost as if in a state of trance, I shut
myself in the house for nine months. I spent the whole day in front of

the television, the days went by, and I kept eating and sleeping. I only went out to go to the cemetery to visit my mother. On the way back, I would stop by the supermarket to buy the foods that at the time were my only consolation: potato chips, Nutella, jam, mayonnaise and sweets of all kinds.

One day, after another of endless quarrels with my sisters, who reproached me for my indifference towards life, I let them convince me to consult a psychologist. With his help I was finally able to understand myself and my anger towards God, who had taken away my mom, but especially my disappointment at not having been able to tell her how much I loved her despite our disagreements. The therapy lasted a long time, but after freeing myself from these negative thoughts, I found myself ready to start getting in shape physically.

I had seen plenty of dietologists, and had even spent two months at a specialized institute to treat obesity, but then I gained weight again and the scale pointed once more past the one hundred kilogram mark. I have always felt like a chunk of meat.

By chance one day I met a girl who told me she had lost 30 kilos without taking any pills. It took me a moment to recognize her as a former co-worker of mine! She had always been heavy, but now she was gorgeous, with a relaxed face and obvious enthusiasm. I had her give me your telephone number and I got in touch with you. Before, I never managed to stick to a diet for more than a week, after which I felt I was going crazy and started eating even more than before. I realized that the decision to change my looks radically had to come from inside me, and I eventually reached a point where I had the courage to tell myself the time had now come to make a definite change in my life.

The first time I came to your office, I thought it would surely be like any other visit, but instead you made me feel like I was unique. You explained many aspects relating to my problem, and strongly reassured me.

Even if only the dietary therapy would have brought positive results, I nonetheless needed to be helped, because by myself I was not capable of sticking to a diet.

I remember that I told you, the first time I saw you, 'Doctor, please help me lose weight, and scold me if I don't listen'.

You made me feel at ease, since you didn't see me as a fat person. I understood this because whatever questions I asked you about the diet or my physical appearance, you gave me answers that showed me my mistakes and allowed me to analyze myself.

Psychologically, I felt assisted. I felt I was not alone, and this helped me be more motivated.

When I went home I told my boyfriend and my sisters how enthusiastic I was. Your answers were always very positive. I remember that when I asked you if I could get down to a size 44, which I wore when I was fourteen, you reassured me and instilled confidence in me. Even if I had doubts about my own willpower, you made me feel confident and encouraged me to do better.

I met my boyfriend when I was on the diet you prescribed for me. I had already lost over 20 kilos. He was attracted by my easy-going, natural attitude. In fact, while I was losing weight my character began to change; I became more cheerful and gained self-confidence. Even if I still had some weight to lose, I knew that you were there and that I would surely make it happen.

Caption pg, 139

THE DOCTOR'S ROL

When following a diet, patients trust in the doctor's authority. It's as if they returned to being like a child, when their parents made the decisions, and guided and scolded them.

My boyfriend helped me psychologically; he was even willing to not go out to eat so I could stick to my diet. He would call me, asking me whether I had followed your dietary advice and done the exercises you had instructed me to do, such as the step, and how long I had done them. He spurred me on, insisting: 'You need to keep going, you can't give up, keep going.' That way I looked in the mirror and I told my reflection: 'You can do it'."

The medical treatment

Diet

My patient had a problem with hypercholesterolemia (high choles-terol), with values around 250 mg/dl. Her mother had died of a heart attack and Marinella feared she was at risk too.

Since in her diet she was allowed only a little pasta, and she felt the need for more, I advised her to eat a good serving of 120 grams of whole wheat pasta every now and then, topped with a spoonful of oil, fresh tomatoes and Parmesan cheese.

Marinella learned to manage her diet in a personal way by substi-tuting certain foods. For example, to make breaded chicken, she used 100 grams of chicken and ten grams of breadcrumbs and instead of frying it, she baked it in the oven. Thus, little by little, with some cre-ativity she was able to substitute overly repetitive menus.

Even her sisters tried to help out by cooking tasty and low-calorie recipes, and helping her during the hard times. Every now and then I let her eat something not in her diet, to keep her from feeling under too much pressure.

For the first six months I prescribed her an 1800-Calorie diet. she needed this many Calories, because her metabolism was high and her stomach dilated. Marinella was, in fact, accustomed to consuming over 3000 Calories a day.

After this period, because her base metabolism had been lowered by losing

Caption pg. 140 **1800-Calorie diet**

pg. 174-78

weight, for the last four months I gave her a 1400-Calorie diet.

Once my patient had lost 40 kilos, I prescribed her a period of weight maintenance, meaning I allowed her enough Calories to maintain that weight for one month with a 2800-Calorie diet. During the five following months, she could stop following the diet and eat a greater variety of foods.

Six months later we began the diet again to reach her total weight loss goal of 50 kilos, her current weight.

We started with a 900-Calorie diet three times a week, leaving the patient free to consume more Calories on the other four days, as long as she paid attention to what she ate. After two months Marinella reached her goal.

Internal therapy

To reduce her desire for sweet foods and promote the growth of muscle volume, I prescribed her chromium picolinate.

For the water retention, *betulla*.

For her hunger between meals, *ispaghul*.

For the unconscious depression during nocturnal awakenings, ignatia. To disintoxicate the liver and improve its functioning, boldo.

For her morning tiredness, *guarana*.

For the water retention in her legs, *redcurrants*. For the circulation in her legs, *bioflavanoids*. For her dry skin, *beta-carotene*.

Caption pg. 141

1400-Calorie diet pg. 164-68 2800-Calorie diet pg. 179-83
900-Calorie diet
pg. 157-59
Phitotherapy
pg. 184-93
manca pag 148

thighs, mesotherapy on the front of her knees, and mesotherapy combined with ultrasounds on her inner thighs, for a total of 15 sessions.

The change

Marinella confided to me at the end of the therapy how important it had been for her to have someone to guide her in her weight loss program:

"Your help was indispensable for me during the times when everything seemed impossible. Your precise instructions always showed me a way out and gave me hope.

Now, at age 31, after one and a half years, I finally weigh 50 kilos less. I feel born again and am making up for lost time, as if I had been released from a prison of fat."

Now she is sure of herself. Certainly, having succeeded in reaching a major goal has helped her get a new perspective on life.

"Ever since I lost weight, I have ceased to be afraid of the future. You made me feel like reaching my goal. You're so enthusiastic about your work that you communicated your excitement to me, and I couldn't let you down! I wasn't this committed for myself alone, but also because I know it means a lot to you. I'm sure you would have appreciated me even if I hadn't seen these results. This is your work, and you give so much of yourself because you really care about your patients' problems, otherwise you wouldn't do what you do."

I was pleasantly surprised by these flattering comments and was happy when she shared with me how she'd changed inside.

"Now I feel much more energetic and determined than ever before, I want to be heard.

I am also more neurotic, but I go out now, go dancing, stay out late with friends,

BEING THIN AND FEELING GREAT

Anger is a normal response to situations that seek to efface the personality of an individual. Obese people tend to conceal such feelings towards others, dealing with them instead by eating enormous quantities of food. When a person loses weight their self-esteem increases and, consequently, so does their ability to deal with the outside world in a more assertive way.

and am not ashamed anymore when others looks at me, because I think I look rather pretty; many people say so. Now I can look at myself in a mirror again without rejecting the image it reflects.

My relationships with others have changed. Now I speak up for myself and if I get angry, I deal with the situation head on. I feel very different ever since I lost weight. I have a different relationship with myself; before it was as if the fat suffocated the real me. People who are thin cannot understand what it feels like to be oppressed by an excess of 50 kilos.

But now the situation has reversed. I am psychologically stronger and I feel like there is something wonderful inside me about to explode. I feel like I can change anything I get my hands on for the better, face any situation and succeed in any project. In the mirror I do not see a thin, pretty person; I just see myself, and this gives me great strength.

Now I long to live with my boyfriend; before I didn't even have a boyfriend, and there was no one with whom I might want to live."

Part Three

Self-help treatment
Dealing with your own situation

How to diagnose your problem

Before looking for a possible solution to your cellulite, it is absolutely essential to understand to what extent the cellulite has developed.

Self-examination

Stand in front of a mirror and observe your thighs and legs carefully.

If your skin is lumpy and you are at your ideal weight or overweight, it is possible that you have *third* or *fourth stage* cellulite.

In this case, it is better to consult a specialist experienced in treating cellulite.

If, instead, your skin is taught, pale, and has nodules when pinched, we are probably dealing with *second-third-stage* cellulite.

In this case, the help of a specialist is not always necessary; you can even begin treating it yourself at home.

A medical diagnosis

The best method for determining to what extent cellulite has developed is, of course, to see a specialist who can give you a more precise idea as to how to deal with this 'enemy'.

A doctor, in order to make a diagnosis, uses the following methods: *inspection, palpation, thermography* and *impedance analysis.*

INSPECTION

Enables the external appearance of the skin to be analyzed, checking for capillaries or stretch marks and the condition of the veins, especially in the legs.

PALPATION

Is used to determine the texture of the skin, and to detect the presence and consistency of cellulite nodules, by feeling the skin.

USE THESE QUESTIONS TO BETTER DEFINE YOUR GOALS
Answer with absolute sincerity!
IS THERE SOMETHING YOU WOULD LIKE TO DO BUT ARE NOT DOING?

WHAT ARE YOUR REASONS FOR LOSING WEIGHT?
o Improve your overall health
o Breathe easier
o Be able to go up stairs without panting
o Others

AT WHAT WEIGHT DID YOU REALLY FEEL IN SHAPE?
IN WHAT TIME FRAME WOULD YOU LIKE TO REACH THIS WEIGHT?
WHAT ARE YOUR FAVORITE ACTIVITIES?
U Go shopping Ll Do hobbies
o Talk with friends
o Phone a loved one
o Go see a movie
o Listen to music
o Dancing
o Physical activity
o Others: what?
AT WHAT WEIGHT DID YOU REALLY FEEL IN SHAPE?
THERMOGRAPHY
THERMOGRAPHY The doctor uses a strip of cholesterol crystal which shows a variation in color according to the heat emitted by the skin. The areas in which the greatest amount of cellulite is found are cooler, since less blood (which is warm) circulates through it. The tem-

perature differences are shown on the surface of the test strip by an array of colors ranging from blue, which indicates the absence of cellulite, to black, indicating the presence of a serious condition with fibrosis and circulatory distress. The intermediate colors are green—which indicates lymphatic stagnation—and brown—indicating fibrosis in process.

IMPEDANCE ANALYSIS In addition to such techniques for diagnosis, impedance analysis helps the doctor to visualize the patient's body composition and to quantify the fat and muscle tissue.
mu muscle tissue.

OUR BODY AND ITS RESISTANCE TO ELECTRIC ENERGY
The concept of impedance is based on the principle that the body, due to its ionic conformation, resists the passage of sinusoidal electric currents.

The electric conductivity of the body is linked to its ionic component and is proportional to the free ions found in salts, bases and acids. Muscle tissue in particular contains a large quantity of water and electrolytes and is therefore an excellent conductor; fat and bones, however, are dielectric tissues, and are therefore poor conductors. Usually, the adhesive electrodes are attached to the right hand and foot. The patient must not have eaten for at least four hours, have a hydro-electrolytic balance and remain lying on his back with legs together during the test.

It will be necessary to distinguish between the therapies suitable for the first and second stages and those required for the other two types, especially in cases of third and fourth degree cellulite, since these are the most serious types and the therapy, if not conducted properly, might aggravate them.

How to solve the problem of cellulite in the first and second stages

DIET

The first rule to follow is to have a balanced diet and to reduce the amount of salt consumed, which causes water retention. Nevertheless, it is important to remember that people with low blood pressure (hypotension) must not eliminate salt completely from their diet, because this could cause tiredness and, in extreme cases, fainting (lipothymia), especially during the summer months, when we lose more minerals from sweating.

All fried foods must be eliminated, since they slow down digestion and are much higher in calories than boiled or steamed foods. Moreover, frying food also produces free radicals, substances responsible for the aging of the skin and the hardening of the capillaries.

An excess of Calories leads to an increase in weight and, in the case of a gynoid type build, in which the adipose tissue accumulates in the lower section of the body, the excess kilos will settle in the upper thigh area (trochanteric region).

Naturally, all kinds of vegetables are recommended, because they contain between 20 and 60 Calories on average per 100 grams, and therefore eating large quantities of vegetables does not carry any risks as long as only a little oil or dressing is added to them. One spoonful of oil contains 90 Calories, so it is easy to increase one's calorie intake without realizing it.

Foods like pasta, bread, gnocchi, rice and polenta (cornmeal) can be eaten in servings of up to 150 grams per day, according to one's daily calorie requirements. It is simply important to not overdo it with the sauces and toppings, which are high in fat.

PHYSICAL EXERCISE

Exercises, running, athletics and most sports in general are allowed. The ideal situation would be to get at least one hour of exercise per day, at any age.

Those who have little free time can walk at least one hour a day, even splitting up their exercise time throughout the day (for example, 10-15 minutes in the morning, and 20 minutes after lunch and dinner), so as to avoid lymphatic

Caption pg. 149

WHAT EXERCISES?
The most suitable ones are stretching exercises. They lengthen the muscles and squeeze them, so the liquids can be absorbed.

retention and allow the body to eliminate toxins.

Getting some exercise after eating allows more calories to be used up, and 10 minutes of exercise after the evening meal make us sleepy and help us to relax.

The benefits obtained by getting regular physical exercise include:—reduction of body fat,

—increase in lean body mass,—lower blood pressure,

—lower risk of osteoporosis (which is always on the lurk after menopause),—reduced stress and slowdown of aging processes.

To lose one kilo, the body must burn 7000 Calories. By walking briskly about 250 Calories are consumed in one hour, which is not a lot; this is why exercising alone is not enough to lose weight and must be combined with a diet.

ANTICELLULITE CREAMS

All kinds of anticellulite creams containing substances that help eliminate liquids and strengthen the capillaries can be utilized. It is best to use creams containing *horse-chestnut, butcher's broom, escina* and *caffeine,* and even better if they're combined in phospholipid complexes, which allow the active ingredients to penetrate better. These products increase the blood circulation in the veins and capillaries, strengthen the capillary endothelium and contribute to stimulating the absorption of interstitial liquids.

When applying the cream, you must massage the affected area to stimulate local circulation. The advantages of these creams are also psychological, because it means you are taking take of your body, after perhaps having neglected it for a long time.

PLASTIFIED WARM-UP SUIT

You may want to slip on a plastified warm-up suit before going jogging and in this way eliminate excess liquids.

Under the plastic leggings it is important to wear cotton tights that can absorb the

Caption pg. 150

THE EFFECTS OF A SEDENTARY LIFESTYLE

Water retention, also caused by a sedentary lifestyle, can lead to the formation of cellulite

liquid lost while running; after exercising, the tights must be removed promptly. Once you have taken a shower, you can apply the anticellulite cream.

SALT WATER BATH

Twice a week you can add a kilo of coarse salt to your bathwater and soak in it for at least 30 minutes. Afterwards you will feel a pleasant sensation of reduced swelling, since the liquids will pass by osmosis to the area of greater saline concentration. The same effect is felt in seawater.

PHYTOTHERAPY

Mildly diuretic herbal teas may help in eliminating the cushions of cellulite, since in many cases medicinal herbs allow the water in the tissue to be drained more effectively. In addition, there are herbal mixes in the form of capsules that provide effective prevention or remedy in the event of edematose cellulite.

DRINKING WATER

Many people drink very little because they're convinced this increases the deposits of cellulite. Actually, drinking mineral water has an excellent effect on the exchange of liquids and is, moreover, essential for eliminating toxins from our body. If they prefer, people may drink herbal teas or fruit and vegetable juice instead. The right amount is at least one liter per day.

COFFEE AND TEA

These two beverages should not be eliminated as they are diuretic, tonic and act as lipolytic agents, which help dissolve fat.

MASSAGES

In order to be effective massages must be performed with delicate, rhythmic, circular movements, starting from the ankles and working up to the top of the thighs, near the lymphatic glands. Massages may be used in combination with other therapies, since they help drain the liquid from tissues and tone up the skin.

Even at a psychological level, they are beneficial since they help us to relax. The massages must nonetheless be done by trained massage therapists, because if they are too rough, they may even break the capillaries and damage the condition of the tissues.

How to solve the problem of cellulite in the third and fourth stages

These two stages call for medical assistance. Violent exercise and massages performed with pounding techniques may even aggravate the problem.

For those with third degree cellulite, walking is not enough, and they will have to undergo treatment of the subcutaneous tissue, in the region affected by cellulite. The fibrous tissue is already developing and only medical therapy will bring a real improvement. Second-degree cellulite, on the other hand, may regress to the first stage only through physical exercise, because the regular motion allows the excess liquid accumulated in the tissues to be drained.

Standing for long periods, in the same position, will make the problem worse.

For those affected instead by cellulite in the fourth stage, it is better if they do not start any exercise classes unless they are undergoing specific medical therapy at the same time. Cellulite at this stage is composed mostly of fibrous tissue, such as that found in scabs, which encapsulates the fat. This cannot be dissolved by frenetic movement, which, on the contrary, may lead to the formation of lactic acid, thus causing even further circulatory damage.

The use of penetrating therapy, such as mesotherapy, enables the medication to reach the cellulite deposits directly, making it easier to dissolve them, which is impossible to achieve by treating them externally.

Of course, if the person is overweight, he/she will have to go on a low-calorie diet, ranging between 900 and 1500 Calories, depending on their base

caption pg. 152

Mesotherapy
pg. 200-01

900-Calorie diet pg. 157-59 1500-Calorie diet pg. 169-73

metabolism (i.e. the number of Calories consumed when lying down and in a state of physical, digestive and emotional relaxation). If the patient is underweight, the therapy will be combined with a high-calorie diet.

Their diet will have to include at least a half-kilo of fruit, for its potassium and vitamin content, particularly for the vitamin C, which protects the capillaries and is found in citus fruits and kiwis, in addition to vegetables, which are rich in minerals and have a diuretic effect, such as asparagus.

Even if it is a person with a normal weight, it will be important for the therapy to be combined with a diet that can limit the formation of free radicals, also partly responsible for the damage to the membranes of adipose cells, eliminating fried foods from their diet.

It should nonetheless not be forgotten that a crash diet, involving a drastic reduction in Calories, is not enough to get rid of those cellulite cushions. This problem, after a large amount of weight is lost, may even get worse, because cellulite is composed not only of adipose tissue, but also of fibrous tissue that has adipose tissue trapped in it. The weight lost from dieting will involve mainly the fat which is easy to lose, located in the breasts, shoulders, arms and face. Therefore, when following a low calorie diet, the weight loss must be gradual; no more than a few hundred grams per week if the person is slightly overweight; and no more than one kilo per week if they need to lose over ten kilos.

Along with the diet, it is essential to treat the problem with localized medical therapies that can act internally, thereby improving the local circulation, breaking up the fibrotic tissue and dissolving the fat.

Obviously, in these cases a personalized therapy that has been carefully studied by a specialized doctor is necessary.

The five most effective kinds of therapy include: *Mesotherapy, Ultrasound therapy, Laser therapy, Magnetic therapy,* and *Electro-toning therapy* (pg. 200-06).

Diets

No treatment that has weight loss as its ultimate goal can preclude dieting, even if it is always necessary to consult a specialist to determine with accuracy which diet is most suited to each individual.

Almost invariably, after someone has gone on a low-calorie diet in which a weight loss of 5% or more was achieved, they will feel more energetic, because they have become more agile. Also, their enthusiasm grows as they see their set goal draw nearer.

To maintain their weight, women generally require 2300 Calories, and men 2900 Calories, with moderate activity.

Advice when following a diet

There are certain hints that are useful to follow if you are on a diet to lose weight. These will make it less difficult to obey the dietologist's advice, since they enable you to personally experience how certain wrong eating behaviors may cause you to gain weight without even realizing it.

EAT meals sitting at the table and not standing. **CHEW** slowly every bite.

AVOID talking while eating so as not to swallow air and to digest better. **PREPARE BEFORE** sitting at the table the amount you want to eat.

AT RESTAURANTS decide beforehand what you will eat; if the first course is large, it is better to eat this with only some vegetables, or take some food off the plate.

DRINK A LITER OF WATER PER DAY, fizzy or not (5 glasses per day). Tea and coffee as often as you like, with moderation if you suffer from hypertension. Plenty of mint, lemon balm, and fruit teas.

IN THE EVENING when cooking dinner or before starting to eat your meal, it is good to drink a cup of vegetable broth prepared with freeze-dried broth, a

(caption pg. 154)

WHAT TO DO IN CASE OF AN ACUTE HUNGER ATTACK
Take note of

a) the time, place and how you felt.
b) the quantity and quality of food you ate.
c) how you felt afterwards.

bouillon cube or fresh vegetables.

IT IS BETTER to use oil from cold-pressed olives on salad and other foods.

USE A TEASPOON OR TABLESPOON as a measuring unit to avoid serving too much dressing.

TOMATO SAUCE may be used to one's liking, either home-cooked or storebought, including the kind with basil (checking to make sure there is no added oil).

TO SEASON your sauces, use all kinds of herbs (rosemary, salvia, thyme, etc...). PICKLED CONSERVES may be eaten to one's liking, (checking to make sure there is no oil).

PREPARE a bowl of celery, carrots and fennel to eat when you feel your stomach grumbling or feel like munching on something (100 gr of fennel=16 Cal.). FRESH FRUIT is essential for its vitamin and fiber content.

VEGETABLES are necessary for their minerals and high fiber content, and they also make you feel full.

AVOID FRIED FOODS as they are very high in calories. SUBSTITUTE sugar with aspartame.

AVOID alcoholic drinks and sweetened beverages. EQUIVALENTS
1 teaspoon of sugar=5 gr

1 tablespoon=10 gr.

WHAT TO DO WHEN YOU CRAVE SWEETS. Women have a pref-
erence for sweet foods, probably because of the estrogen, and men prefer protein foods, apparently because of their testosterone and a
greater amount of muscle tissue. The favorite food of women is chocolate, so as an 'extra food', in case they feel a craving for sweets, I prescribe a bite-size chocolate or a chocolate bar for children once a day. It
contains substances such as theobromine (tonic), magnesium (anti-
stress) and phenylethylamine (which gives us a feeling of comfort).
The sugars and fats contained in chocolate give a certain feeling of
fullness.

For men, instead, I advise two slices of Parma ham and some pickled vegetables if they feel the need to eat between meals.

TO PREPARE A LOW-FAT SAUCE to use on pasta dishes, pour a
can of peeled tomatoes (250 gr) into a pan, add one teaspoon of freeze-
dried vegetable broth, salt to taste, basil, and let simmer for 5 minutes.

When following a diet, it is difficult to make others respect your
desire to eat moderate portions, especially if you have a busy social
life. Here is what to say to avoid every temptation:

1) 'No, thank you, I'm on a diet'. If this is said politely but firmly, the
other person will not insist.

2) Making use of the doctor's judgment: 'My doctor *says this is* not
good for my *health*'. A polite person will leave you alone.

3) I would prefer smaller *portions, so* afterwards I won't feel guilty,
accompanying your statement with a smile of intent.

4) For me food is a drug, so 1 need you to help me control myself. In
any case, I prefer low-fat *foods*.

5) Last night 1 *didn't* feel well, and I'm a bit nauseous. Please *don't*
insist.

6) Lately, I've developed some allergies to some *foods but* am not
sure *which* ones.

GRATIFY YOURSELF WITH A GIFT

For every three kilos lost give yourself a nice present, as long as it's not food. If you feel sad and lonely, switch on the radio or a walkman, raise the volume and dance for at least 10 minutes in front of the mirror. Imagine yourself attractive, sexy and thin at a fantastic party.

If you belong to a fitness club, run over to get some exercise. After a half hour of exercise your <u>organism begins to burn up body fat.</u>

Even though for a diet to be effective it must be based on the individual needs of each patient, you will find on the following pages some examples of diets for varying calorie requirements useful for fighting against the most common problems of cellulite and excess weight. They were drawn up with the Dietosystem program.

900-Calorie diet
(three days)

Day .1
BREAKFAST *PARTIALLY SKIMMED MILK WITH BREAKFAST POWDER Milk 4 0z • Instant breakfast WHOLE WHEAT CRACKERS 1 0z*

LUNCH *FRESH TOMATO SALAD WITHOUT OIL 4 oz+BOILED CHICKEN 4 oz+BREADSTICKS 1 oz KAKI FRUIT 5 oz MINERAL WATER*

DINNER *RICE AND BEAN Rice 1,5 oz • Fresh beans 0,5 oz • Onion * Olive oil (*) • Parmesan cheese a little spoon * Vegetable broth 55 gr* TO PREPARE *In a saucepan brown the onion in a dash of olive oil, add in the beans, some vegetable broth and simmer for about 15 minutes. When cooked combine rice and remaining broth. When the rice has absorbed the liquid, sprinkle with Parmesan. BRAISED LENTILS Lentils 2 spoon • Celery 0,5 oz * Carrots 1 oz • Garlic • Rosemary • Peeled tomatoes 0,5 oz • Olive oil (*)* TO PREPARE

Soak the lentils in slightly salty cold water for at least 12 hours. Rinse and boil them in 112 liter salted water fro an hour and a half. Dice the carrots, celery and onion. In a saucepan cook the vegetables in a dash of oil, add in diced, peeled tomatoes and braise on low heat for about 20 minutes

.one KIWIS WATER

	Protein	Glucides	Lipids	Calories
Calculated requirements	48.53	132.72	24.58	913.05

(*) *Foods with high calorie content. Total daily amount: Olive oil 5 gr*

Day 2
BREAKFAST *PARTIALLY SKIMMED YOGHURT 4 oz MOZZARELLA AND TOMATO SANDWICH Wheat bread 2 oz • Tomato one spoon • Mozzarella 1 oz • Oregano*

LUNCH *SALAD WITH FENNEL AND LEMON Fennel 3 oz • Lemon juice GRILLED SWORDFISH 3 oz ITALIAN BREAD 2 oz, one APPLE WATER*

DINNER *BOILED FENNEL AND LEMON JUICE Fennel 4 oz • Lemon juice CREAM OF PEAS Fresh peas 4 oz • Onion 1 oz • Carrots 1 oz *Lettuce 2 oz • Celery 1 oz • Parmesan cheese 1 spoon • Olive oil (*) TO* PREPARE *Dice all the vegetables and boil in plenty of salted water for about 30 minutes. When cooked, pass through a sieve and top with some olive oil and Parmesan cheese. one BANANA MINERAL WATER*

	Protei	Glucides	Lipids	Calories
Calculated requirements	48.53	132.72	24.58	913.05

(") *Foods with high calorie content. Total daily amount: Olive oil 5 gr*

Day 3
BREAKFAST *PARTIALLY SKIMMED MILK AND
CORNFLAKES Milk 4 oz • Corn flakes 1 oz SOY BREAD
2 oz*

LUNCH *GREEN SALAD Lettuce 3 oz • Olive oil (*) FIL-
LET OF BEEF WITH LEMON Lean beef 3 oz • Lemon
juice 1 little spoon* TO PREPARE *Cook the fillet of beef
on both sides on a griddle for a few minutes. Cover with
lemon juice when done. WHOLE WHEAT BREAD 2 oz,
one PEAR MINERAL WATER*

DINNER *WHOLE GRAIN RICE WITH VEGETABLES Rice 2 oz • Celery
1 oz • Zucchini 1oz • Carrots 1 oz • Onion 1 oz l • Fresh peas 1 oz • Olive
oil (*) • Vegetable broth 3 oz • Parmesan cheese 5 gr* TO PREPARE *In a
sauce pan cook the onion in a little olive oil until golden, add in the celery
and carrots and let simmer a few minutes. Add the zucchini sliced in round
pieces and the peas. After a few minutes, combine rice and broth. Cook for
about 20 minutes. Sprinkle with Parmesan when done. STEAMED BROC-
COLI Broccoli 4 oz h • Lemon juice 5 gr GRAPEFRUIT 200 gr WATER*

	Protein	Glucides	Lipids	Calories
Calculated requirements	48.53	132.72	24.58	913.05

(') *Foods with high caloric content. Total daily amount: Olive oil 10 gr*

1200-Calorie diet
(four days)

Day 1
BREAKFAST
PARTIALLY SKIMMED MILK 5ozr PLAIN COOKIES

LUNCH *POTATO, CARROTAND TOMATO SOUP Potatoes 5 ozr * Peeled tomatoes 1 oz r • Onion 1 oz * Fresh basel • Carrots 3 oz, Parsley • Olive oil (*)* TO PREPARE *Peel and dice the potatoes and carrots, slice the onion, and simmer in a saucepan on low heat with a little water. After 45 minutes, add the peeled tomatoes, and chopped parsley and basel. Cook until the potatoes are slightly mushy, adding some water when necessary and, when done, serve with oil. STEAMED PEAS WITH OIL Fresh peas 4 oz •* Onion 1 oz • Olive oil (*) TO PREPARE *Slice onion and place in a saucepan with a few spoonfuls of water. Cover and cook over low heat. When the onion is soft, add in peas. Add water as necessary and, when done, serve with oil. BANANA one MINERAL WATER*

DINNER *GRILLED DENTEX WITH OIL Dentex 5 oz • Olive oil (*) SALAD WITH* SOY SPROUTS *AND CORN Soy sprouts 3 oz • Celery 1 oz • 1 oz r • Olive oil (*) 3 clementines MINERAL WATER*

Protein	Glucides	Lipids	Calories
calculated requirements	57.90	153.78	38.31	1153.05

(") Foods with high calorie content. Total *daily* amount. Olive oil 25 *gr*

Day 2
BREAKFAST
PARTIALLY SKIMMED MILK 5 oz PLAIN COOKIES 1 oz

LUNCH *SPECIALTY PASTA WITH CHICKPEA SAUCE Specialty pasta 2 oz • Potatoes 1 oz • Dried chickpeas 1oz • Celery 0,5 oz • Onion 0,5 oz • Parmesan 0,5 oz • Olive oil (*)* TO PREPARE *Soak the chickpeas in cold water overnight. Peel all the vegetables, dice and place in a saucepan with the chickpeas and water. Let simmer for about one hour. When done, pass through a sieve, return to pan, add in pasta and cook for 10-15 minutes. Serve with oil and Parmesan. STEAMED SPINACH Spinach 7 oz • Lemon juice • Olive oil (*) ORANGES one MINERAL WATER*

DINNER
*SMOOTH DOGFISH WITH TOMATO dogfish 4 oz; peeled tomatoes 3 oz;
chopped onion and a dash of olive oil, add in the dogfish and cook on moder-
ate head, adding water if necessary.*
MIXED SALAD lettuce 4 oz; fennel 1 oz tomatoes 2 oz; carrots 1 oz; olive oil
TANGERINES 6 oz

Protein	Glucides	Lipids	Calories	
Calculated requirements	57.80	169.26	35.00	1180.91

(*) *Foods with high calorie content. Total daily amount: Olive oil* 20 gr

Day 3
BREAKFAST *PARTIALLY SKIMMED MILK 5 oz r*
PLAIN COOKIES 1 oz

LUNCH *CREAM OF LEGUMES SOUP Fresh beans 4 oz • Carrots 3 oz r
• Onion 1 oz, Zucchini 3 oz • Celery 0,5 oz • Dried chickpeas 0,5 oz
•Parmesan 0,5 oz • Olive oil (*) CRUDITES Carrots 6 oz • Potatoes 2 oz •
Celery 1 oz • Olive oil (') KIWIS two; WATER*

DINNER *DOGFISH WITH PEPPERS Dogfish 5 oz • Onion 0,5 oz •
Fresh garlic, 0, 5 oz • Peppers 3 oz • Vegetable broth 8 oz* TO PREPARE
*Place the fish in a frying pan and the chopped peppers with a few cups of
broth. Add in the onion and a clove of garlic, both chopped, and cook for 10
minutes. TOSSED SALAD Peppers 3 oz • Onion 1 oz r• Tomatoes 1 oz •
Lettuce 1 oz • Olive oil (*) APPLES one; MINERAL WATER*

	Protein	Glucides	Lipids	Calories
Calculated requirements	62.41	156.05	32.84	1130.41

('') *Foods with high calorie content. Total daily amount. Olive oil 15 gr*

Day 4
BREAKFAST *PARTIALLY SKIMMED MILK 5 oz r*
PLAIN COOKIES 1 oz

DINNER *GRILLED TURKEY 4 oz FRESH SALAD Lettuce 2 oz* • *Carrots 1 oz r• Corn 1 oz* • *Lemon juice PINEAPPLE 7 oz MINERAL WATER*

	Protein	Glucides	Lipids	Calories
Calculated requirements	65.58	166.43	34.75	1199.16

(*) *Foods with high calorie content. Total daily amount: Olive oil 10 gr*

LUNCH
CHICKPEA SOUP
   Dried chickpeas 2 oz • Pasta 2,5 oz • Rosemary • Fresh garlic • Olive oil (*) TO PREPARE Soak the chickpeas in lukewarm water with a pinch of baking soda overnight. Drain and boil in a saucepan for about two hours. In a frying pan, cook the chopped garlic in a little oil with the rosemary, pour in the chickpeas and some of the water and simmer for another hour and a half. Add in the pasta and serve immediately when done. CAULIFLOWER SALAD Cauliflower 4 oz • Olive oil (*) PEARS one;WATER

1400-Calorie diet
For lymphatic stagnation (five days)

Dav 1
BREAKFAST
BREAKFAST DRINK WITH PARTIALLY SKIMMED MILK Milk 5 oz •
Breakfast powder 0,5 oz MOZZARELLA AND TOMATO SANDWICH
Wheat bread 1,5 oz • *Tomato 1 0z* • *Mozzarella 1 oz* • *Oregano*
SNACK; *GRAPEFRUIT one*

LUNCH *GRILLED LEAN BEEF 4 oz CARROTS, POTATOES AND ZUCCHINI Carrots 4 oz • Potatoes 2 oz• Zucchini 2 oz • Lemon juice one teaspoon • Olive oil (*) CRACKERS 1 oz ; WATER*

SNACK *KIWI one*

DINNE*MACARONI WITH TOMATO SAUCE Macaroni 2 oz • Peeled tomatoes 2 oz • Parmesan 0,5 oz • Olive oil (*) • Onion 0,5 oz • Fresh basil leaves* TO PREPARE *Brown the onion in a dash of oil, add in tomatoes and cook for about 20 minutes, then pour over the pasta. Add flavor with a few fresh basil leaves.* OCTOPUS WITH GARLIC *Octopus 4 oz • Garlic, one clove • Green pepper • Parsely • Olive oil (*)* TO PREPARE *Use even frozen octopus. After cleaning it, place in a saucepan with the oil, one clove of garlic, whole or chopped, and the pepper. Cover, placing a sheet of paper under the lid, and cook on low heat for about half an hour. Add salt when done.* FENNEL, POTATOES AND CARROTS *Fennel 5 oz • Carrots 2 oz • Potatoes 2 oz • Olive oil (*)* MINERAL WATER

Protein	Glucides	Lipids	Calories	
Calculated requirements	73.57	208.82	43.52	1469.00

(") *Foods with high calorie content. Total daily amount: Olive oil 25 gr*

Day 2

BREAKFAST *PARTIALLY SKIMMED MILK WITH COFFEE Milk 5 oz • Coffee 1 oz CRACKERS AND MOZZARELLA Crackers 1 oz • Fresh mozzarella 0,5 oz*

SNACK *APPLE one*

LUNCH *BEEF CUTLETS WITH ROSEMARY Lean beef 4 oz • Garlic, one clover • Olive oil (*) •Rosemary* TO PREPARE *Pour a little water in a skillet, add the garlic and the beef sprinkled with rosemary. Cook on low heat and before taking it off the heat add the olive oil.* MEDITERRANEAN PEPPERS *Peppers 4 oz * Peeled tomatoes 1 oz r* TO PREPARE *Roast the pep-*

pers slightly, peel off the skin and cut in slices. Cook on low heat in a skillet with the tomatoes. Season with pepper, salt and oregano. WHEAT BREAD 2 *oz gr* WATER

SNACK *BAKED PEARS Pears one* • *Sugar (*)*
DINNER *BOILED RICE 2 oz* PORK CHOP WITH OIL *Lean pork 2 oz* • *Olive oil (*)* TO PREPARE *Cook the pork chop in a hot skillet on both sides for about 8-10 minutes. When done season with a dash of olive oil.* GRATED CARROTS WITH OIL *Carrots 5 oz* • *Olive oil (*)a Lemon juice one teapoon* MINERAL WATER

Protein	Glucides	Lipids	Calories
73,57	208,82	43,52	1469.00

(") Foods with high calorie content.
Total daily amount. Olive oil 2 spoon / Sugar 1 spoon

Day 3
BREAKFAST *PARTIALLY SKIMMED MILK 5 oz* TOASTED BREAD WITH RICOTTA *Toasted bread 1 oz* • *Fresh ricotta 1 oz*

SNACK *PEARS one*
LUNCH *TURKEY BREAST WITH HERBS Turkey breast 3 oz* • *Carrots 0,5 oz r* • *Celery 0,5 oz* • *Olive oil (*)* • *Rosemary* TO PREPARE *Boil the turkey with the carrot and celery. Add the oil, rosemary and lemon juice, and let simmer on low heat until done. Salt and pepper if allowed.* PEPPERS AND TOMATOES *Peppers 3 oz* • *Peeled tomatoes 3 oz* • *Olive oil (*)* TO PREPARE *Cook the largely chopped peppers with the tomatoes on low heat. Cover the pan. When done add oil and salt if allowed.* WHEAT BREAD 2 *oz* /WATER
SNACK *BAKED APPLES Apple 6 oz* • *Sugar ("')*
DINNER *NOODLES WITH TOMATO AND BASIL SAUCE Noodles 2 oz* • *Peeled tomatoes 3 oz* * *Parmesan 5 gr* • *Olive oil (*)* • *Fresh basil leaves* • *Onion 5 gr* TO PREPARE *Brown the chopped onion in a bit of oil, add the*

tomatoes and cook for 18-20 minutes. Boil the noodles in plenty of salty water, drain, and add in the sauce, some chopped basil leaves and the Parmesan. **MACKEREL AU GRATIN** Mackerel 2 oz • Tomatoes 1 oz * Bay leaves • Olive oil (*)• Fresh parsely * Bread crumbs TO PREPARE Boil the fish. Clean it and place in a greased pan, season with herbs, the diced tomatoes, and bread crumbs. Salt if permitted. Bake for about 30 minutes. Season with oil. TOMATO SALAD WITHOUT OIL 6 oz MINERAL WATER

Protein	Glucides	Lipids		Calories
Calculated requirements	73.57	208.82	43.52	1469.00

(") Foods with high calorie content.
Total daily amount: Olive oil 20 gr / Sugar 10 gr

Day 4
BREAKFAST 'CHOCOLATE' MILK Skimmed milk 5 oz • Cocoa substitute 0,5 oz WHOLE WHEAT CRACKERS 1 oz
SNACK CLEMENTINES three
LUNCH ROASTED CHICKEN 4 oz BOILED CARROTS WITH LEMON JUICE Carrots 6 oz • Lemon juice ITALIAN BREAD 2 oz MINERAL WATER
SNACK GRAPEFRUIT one

DINNER SPAGHETTI WITH TUNAFISH SAUCE Spaghetti 3 oz • Canned tuna fish, partially drained 1 oz • Olive oil (*) • Parsley• Garlic, one clove TO PREPARE Brown the garlic in the oil and throw it away, add in the chunks of tuna fish and let it simmer a few minutes. Boil the spaghetti in plenty of salty water, drain the water and pour the sauce and chopped fresh parsley over it. BAKED SARDINAS Sardinas 3 oz • Bread crumbs 0,5 oz • Olive oil (*) • Rosemary • Vinegar *Lemon juice 3 oz TO PREPARE Marinate the sardines in the vinegar for about half an hour. Rinse them, and coat in bread crumbs, place in a baking pan and cook in the oven. Prepare a sauce with oil, rosemary and lemon juice. Season the fish. GREEN SALAD

WITHOUT OIL Radicchio 3 oz • Belgian endive 1 oz • Escarole 2 oz
WATER

Protein 73,57   Glucides 208,83   Lipids43,52   Calories 1469,00

(*) *Foods with high calorie content. Total daily amount: Olive oil 10 gr*

Day 5
BREAKFAST *PARTIALLY SKIMMED MILK WITH BREAKFAST POW-*
DER Milk 5 oz • Breakfast powder 0,5 oz SOY BREAD 2 oz

SNACK *KIWI two*
LUNCH *STEAMED SALMON Fresh salmon 3 oz r • Lemon juice 0,5oz•*
Olive oil (*) • Parsley TO PREPARE Cook the fish in a little water. Drain
and season with oil, lemon and parsley. BOILED ZUCCHINI WITHOUT
OIL Zucchini 7 oz • Lemon juice ITALIAN BREAD 2 oz WATER
SNACK *BAKED PEARS Pear one • Sugar (*)*
DINNER *SPECIALTY PASTA WITH TURNIP TOPS Specialty pasta 2 oz*
• Turnip tops 2 oz • Olive oil (*) • Parmesan 0,5 • Garlic TO PREPARE
Boil the turnip tops in plenty of salty water, drain and season with pressed
garlic. Meanwhile, cook the pasta and, when done, add in the turnip tops, oil
and Parmesan. BOILED SHRIMP 4 oz POTATOES AND CARROTS
WITH OIL Potatoes 4 oz • Carrots 2 oz • Olive oil (*) MINERAL WATER

	Protein	Glucides	Lipids	Calories
Calculated requirements	73.57	208.82	43.52	1469.00

(*) *Foods with high calorie content.*
Total daily amount: Olive oil 20 gr / Sugar 10 gr

Phytotherapy

Phytotherapy (therapy with plants) stimulates the organism to react
to illnesses, without causing the side effects typical of traditional med-

icine. Naturally, even plants (seeds, roots, leaves or flowers) must be prescribed with caution (in the form of a tincture, powder, glyceric macerato, dry extract, titrate).

When describing the various cases (pg. 62-144), we did not specify in what form and in what quantities the prescribed plants had to be taken, because every individual requires a personalized prescription, which usually varies over the course of therapy.

Principal plants used in phytotherapy

WITCH HAZEL
Is rich in tannins and is an excellent vasoconstrictor for the veins; it is therefore recommended for people who suffer from fragile capillaries, hemorrhoids, varicose veins, phlebitis and circulatory problems in general.

PINEAPPLE
Is considered the ultimate anti-cellulite plant due to its bromelain content—found only in the stem and not in the fruit—which has the property of dissolving the collagen fiber in cellulite and eliminating edema. It is also used for its diuretic and anti-inflammatory effect.

ANGELICA
The root of this plant, used in phytotherapy, contains coumarins and firocoumarins, particularly useful for their antispasmodic and bile-stimulating properties. It is recommended especially for digestive problems, colitis and meteorism.

BETULA
Contains betulin, a substance with a strong diuretic effect, and flavonoids, which have a draining effect on peripheral edema and strengthen the blood vessels. It is useful in cases of kidney stones, water retention and gout.

Caption pg. 184

SENNA, BUT WITH MODERATION

It is important not to exaggerate in the use of plant laxatives, in particular with senna, which irritates the intestines and can **lead to chronic colitis, if not discontinued,** *or of algae products rich in iodine, used both for losing weight and as a laxative, which when taken for a prolonged period—over six months—may lead to thyroid trouble. The latter at* **first increases its function, but** *then due to a regulatory mechanism—Wolf—Chaikoff effect—reduces its activity.*

HAWTHORN

Due to the synergy of flavonoids contained in this plant, hawthorn regulates cardiac frequency, improves coronary circulation and lowers blood pressure. It is also a cardiotonic, reduces palpitations and calms anxiety.

BOLDO

Boldine, found in this plant, stimulates bile production and is useful in liver insufficiency and for gallstones. It also helps overcome digestive problems.

CAMEDRIO

This plant, also called the fat-eating plant, contains tannins and flavonoids, which limit the amount of sugars and fats assimilated. It is a diuretic and accelerates the metabolism (but in high doses may be toxic). It is recommended in weight-loss therapies.

CARBONE VEGETALE

This is used in cases of meteorism for its high capacity to absorb gas, and the bacteria it produces, thereby reducing considerably intestinal fermentation, flatulence and abdominal bloatedness.

ARTICHOKE
This plant, whose active ingredient is concentrated mainly in the leaves, helps reduce cholesterol and fluidifies bile. It is also recommended for stimulating the digestive system in general.

MILK THISTLE
Its active ingredient, silimarine, makes it an effective protector of the liver. It is recommended for difficult digestion and for all types of liver disease (alcoholic, toxic-metabolic, iatrogenic and chronic).

CENTELLA ASIATICA
This plant is utilized to improve the blood circulation, in anticellulite treatments and for fragile capillaries.

CHICORY
The root of this plant is known for its laxative, hypoglycemic and diuretic properties. It is used to prevent drowsiness after meals and to diminish postprandial glycemia.

CYPRESS
Contains tannins, flavonoids and glycolic acid. It is a vasoconstrictor, useful in all types of troubles with the veins. It fights against swollenness in the legs and capillary fragility.

CUMMIN
The fruit of cumin is used for its gastrointestinal regulatory properties. It aids digestion and helps against aerophagy and meteorism.

CALIFORNIA POPPY
It has sedative and hypnotic properties, without causing tolerance and addiction. It reduces the time required to fall asleep and improves the quality of sleep. It is rich in zinc and is also used in case of nervousness, anxiety, depression, headache, itching and urticaria.

GUAR FLOUR

Guar has a hypoglycemic effect and is also used because it gives a feeling of satiety. It is acts as a tonic.

FENNEL

Its active ingredients are trans-aneto! fenchone, estragole and alphaphellandrene. It is used because it stimulates gastrointestinal motility and has a secretionary action in the respiratory tract. It helps against meteorism, bloatedness in the stomach, intestinal spasms and phlogosis of the upper respiratory tract. It is also recommended for colitis, difficult digestion and aerophagy.

ORANGE BLOSSOMS

Rich in flavonoids and vitamins, they have an antispasmic and sedative action and are utilized in cases of anxiety; they also help digestion.

FRANGULA

The rind of this plant has an effective laxative and regulatory effect on the intestines, if the advised doses are respected.

ASH WOOD

This plant has diuretic, laxative, and antirheumatic properties, helps prevent gout and lowers hyperuricemia. It is also used for water retention and edema, and therefore in against cellulite therapy.

FUCUS

The main function of this marine algae is to accelerate metabolism, even if it should be used with moderation due to its high iodine content. It acts on the thyroid, stimulating it initially, but then causes a functional slowdown as a result of the Wolf-Chaikoff effect.

GARCINIA CAMBOGIA

From the rind of this tropical fruit an extract is obtained that is rich in hydroxycitric acid and used in cases of obesity, high cholesterol and triglycerides in the blood, because it intervenes in the metabolism of fats.

GINKGO BILOBA

The leaves of this plant are used because they are rich in flavonoids and bioflavonoids. They stimulate the blood circulation and act against cerebral circulatory disorders, artereosclerosis and free radicals; this is why they are considered excellent for the elderly.

GINSENG

This legendary plant, which has a reputation of being an elixir of long life, is rich in vitamins, amino acids, and estrogens. It has a tonic and revitalizing action, and is used in cases of depression and fatigue. It should be avoided by those suffering from hypertension, since it may raise blood pressure.

GLUCOMANNANO

Is a dried root which on contact with water immediately swells up to 60 times its initial volume, forming a neutral plant gel. This gives a feeling a fullness to the stomach. In addition to providing a good dose of fiber, which offsets constipation, it slows down and reduces the assimilation of glucides and lipids, thus lowering the cholesterol level in the blood.

BERMUDA GRASS

This herb is rich in potassium, vitamins and essential oils. It is a diuretic, has an anti-inflammatory effect on the urinary tract and is recommended in cases of high blood pressure and to reduce edemas.

GUARANA

Using the seeds of this plant, a paste is obtained that is rich in tannin, caffeine, vitamins and minerals, used as a tonic and a stimulant in case of tiredness and weakness; moreover, guarana increases our resistance to hunger stimuli and for this reason is used in cases of obesity and weight-loss diets.

IGNATIA
Is a homeopathic product used to treat exogenous depression and hysteric aphonia.

HORSE CHESTNUT
The seeds and stem of this plant have hiebotonic and vasoprotective properties and is used to treat weak capillaries—on which it has an anti inflammatory and antiedema effect—heavy legs, and in cases of venous insufficiency.

ISPAGHUL
Also called Plantago ovata, it is rich in mucilages and, on contact with water and gastric secretions, swells about 100 times its size creating a non-iritating and non-digestible gel. This gives a sense of fullness, aids intestinal transit and slows down the absorption of food, so it is recommended for weight control purposes. It is also useful in reducing hyperglycemic peaks and for constipation.

LAVENDER
This strongly scented plant is used as a sedative and antispasmodic medicine, and to treat nervousness, light cases of insomnia and infections of the respiratory and urinary tracts. It can also be used in cases of gastrointestinal problems caused by nervousness.

LICORICE
The roots of this plant aid digestion and are used for irritations in the digestive system (gastritis, colics) and in the respiratory system (cough, hoarseness). Persons with high blood pressure and water retention should not take too much of it, because large doses can induce a rise in the blood pressure.

HOP

The bitter and tonic properties of this plant are used in the production of beer, and are what give its bitter aroma. It has sedative and and relaxing effect, aids digestion, and is used for menstrual pain and discomfort during menopause.

LYMPHOMYOSOT

Is a homeopathic product recommended for lymphatic drainage and disintoxication of the liver. It is used to help the liver, which during a diet is put under greater pressure.

MALLOW

Rich in mucilages, this plant is useful for its emollient and anti inflammatory properties in the mucous in the oral cavity, and in the respiratory and gastrointestinal tract. It regulates the intestine and reduces the problems associated with an irritable colon.

LEMON BALM

This plant is effective against spasmodic colitis and an irritable colon, anxiety and nervousness. It is used in cases of insomnia, stress, and to reduce nervous hunger.

MINT

Its leaves have antiseptic, antispasmodic and digestive properties. It is recommended in cases of colitis associated with with abdominal cramps, intestinal fermentation and meteorism.

MILFOIL

Has spasmolytic properties in the digestive system and uterine, and for this reason is used to regulate the menstrual period, lessening the mentrual flow and cramps. It also has sedative and anti inflammatory effects.

OLIVE

This typically Mediterranean plant is used in cases of diabetes and hypertension, because it regulates the blood pressure and has a hypoglycemic effect. Moreover, it has febrifuge properties, recognized since ancient times, and contributes to lowering the 'bad' cholesterol (LDL) and increasing the 'good' cholesterol (HDL).

STINGING NETTLE

This herb, considered as 'nasty' and bothersome, actually has numerous therapeutic properties. It is rich in minerals and vitamins, making it a good remineralizing tonic, and is also effective in reducing the glycemia in the blood, is diuretic, cleanses the liver and helps against intestinal inflammations.

ORTOSIFON

This exotic plant has diuretic and depurative properties. Due to its active ingredients, flavones and potassium salts, it is also a 'fat-burning' plant, and is an adjuvant in weight loss diets.

PAPAYA

Very rich in vitamins (A, C and P) and enzymes, this tropical fruit is useful in cases of digestive problems and flatulence. Its active ingredient, papain, is highly useful in weight loss therapy for people who have widespread and painful cellulite.

PASSIONFLOWER

This plant, which was cultivated by the Aztecs, is recommended in cases of stress, nervousness and anxiety. It reduces anxiety and aids against insomnia, lengthening the amount of sleeping time.

PILOSELLA

Rich in flavonoids and tannins, it has a draining, depurative and diuretic action that makes it very effective in weight loss diets, in treating cellulite and in cases of edema and water retention.

PISCIDIA

This plant, from the Leguminosae family, has diuretic and sedative properties.

BLACKCURRANT

The leaf of this plant, known for its delicious fruit, is used as an adrenocortical stimulant and a general anti-inflammatory. It is diuretic, useful when there is water retention, and helpful in weight loss and cellulite therapy, since it has a depurative effect and protects the capillaries.

ROSA CANINA

Rich in tannins, vitamins and flavonoids, *rosa canina*, otherwise known as dogrose, reinforces the immune system and is an antioxidant. It is recommended for stress, gingivitis, cystitis, diarrhea, and in preventing bacterial infections.

ROSEMARY

This Mediterranean plant, often used for cooking, is an excellent vasoconstrictor and is used as a depurant for the liver and in cases of intestinal pain. It acts as a general tonic and antioxidant. It tends to make the blood pressure rise, and should be administered with caution in cases of hypertension.

RUSCUS

Better known as butcher's broom, it contains r sems, saponins and tannins. eating the berries causes gastrointestinal trouble, but administering the active ingredient reduces the fragility of the capillaries, and consequently, the pain and heaviness in the legs. Due to its effect on the lining of the blood vessels, it improves circulation and tends to alleviate the swelling caused by water retention and the nighttime cramps.

SEPIA COMPOSITUM

Is a homeopathic product, recommended for stress, nervousness and all forms of anxiety.

TARAXACUM

Also called dandelion, it is used in liver insufficiency, and liver disorders of various kinds. It is a diuretic, colagogue (i.e. stimulates bile secretion, essential for the intestinal absorption of lipids) and is also used for constipation, high cholesterol and triglycerides in the blood, besides being an adjuvant in treating cellulite.

GREEN TEA

Has a strong diuretic effect and contains xanthinic bases (caffeine), which have lipolytic properties—i.e. they help dissolve and eliminate fat—and for this reason may be used very effectively in weight loss diets. It is a tonic and acts against free radicals (one cup contains the daily dose of selenium).

THYME

This scented bush used mainly for its antiseptic qualities is helpful in curing gastrointestinal and lung illnesses. It also acts as a tonic, and a diuretic, and counteracts intestinal fermentation.

VALERIAN

One of the best natural tranquilizers, it diminishes anxiousness and reduces the time needed to fall asleep, improving the quality of sleep. It is also helpful for symptoms accompanying menopause (heat flashes, tachycardia, mood swings).

RED BRYONY

Rich in tannins and flavonoids, it is effective against all forms of capillary fragility and circulatory problems in the veins (heavy legs, varicose veins), since it fights against edemas and inflammation. It diminishes menopaus-rerelated troubles, and seems to increase the estrogen levels during menopause.

Herbal teas

Traditionally, plants were used in herbal teas or infusions. Nowadays, modern phytotherapy offers a more practical and concentrated form with herbal powders in capsules. They are easier to use and to swallow. For those who wish to use traditional methods, here are a few examples of herbal teas and their use.

HERBAL TEA FOR CONSTIPATION
Frangula 30 gr • Lemon balm 30 gr • Fennel 30 gr TO PREPARE One spoonful of this mixture for 114 liter of water. Boil for three minutes, let stand for ten, then filter. Drink in the evening warm or lukewarm. The intestines return to normal after two weeks.

HERBAL TEA FOR A BLOATED ABDOMEN
Anise 30 gr • Fennel 30 gr • Cumin 30 gr TO PREPARE One spoonful of this mixture for 250 cl of water. Boil for three minutes, let stand for ten, then filter. Drink after the evening meal.
HERBAL TEA TO AID DIURESIS Taraxacum root 30 gr • Bermuda grass 30 gr • Chicory 30 gr TO PREPARE One spoonful of this mixture of roots for 112 liter of cold water. Bring to a boil, remove from heat and let stand for a few minutes. Drink throughout the day.
HERBAL TEA TO AID DIGESTION AND PREVENT BLOATEDNESS AFTER MEALS Lemon balm 30 gr • Fennel 30 gr • Cummin 30 gr • Angelica 30 gr TO PREPARE One level spoonful of this mixture for 114 liter of water. Boil the water, pour it over the crushed herbs and let stand for 5 minutes. Strain and drink while the infusion is still warm after main meals.

Exercises

Over and beyond the specific instructions and therapies that should be followed, exercise is essential for anyone who seriously intends to lose weight. Floor exercises are ideal even for the laziest of us, because it tones up and strengthens the body without putting too much effort on the lower limbs, often already suffering from the excess adipose tissue and edema. Moreover, the use of special exercise machines can help tone up the parts of the body generally unaccustomed to movement, such as the inner thighs.

Below, you will find some examples of low-impact exercises, suitable for everyone.

The most important rule, however, is to start exercising with a smile; you will discover that, even if you're in a bad mood, this will change quickly.

Revitalizing exercise

Useful for those who sit for long hours at work and want to do a simple exercise to firm up the abdomen and buttocks, tone up the breasts and get rid of psychological stress as a result of sitting too much.

1) Stand with your legs apart and arms raised, keeping your arms and legs aligned.

2) Bend over, with your arms hanging down so as to touch the floor with the tip of your fingers.

This exercise will feel very relaxing if you breathe in deeply while raising your arms, and breathe out energetically while letting your arms hang down to the floor. Repeat this exercise 30 times and it will produce a pleasant feeling of euphoria.

Exercise for inner thighs

1) Stretched out on your side, breathe in while you lift your legs one at a time at right angles, keeping them straight.
2) Breathing out, lower your leg again to the starting position.
Repeat the exercise 5 times until you can work up to 30 leg-lifts.

Exercise for abdomen and thighs

1) Breathing in, lift your legs up without bending your knees until the points of your feet touch the floor behind your head. (If you are not used to stretchng, stop in the position—even 10 cm above the floor—in which you are able to keep your legs straight).
2) Breathe out while you lower your legs to the starting position.
Repeat this exercise 5 times until you can work up to 30 times a day. Every week repeat it three more times.

Exercise for buttocks, thighs and shoulders

It is extremely simple but effective, ideal for everyone. It must be carried out very, very slowly. Before starting it is good to relax.
1) Lying on your back, breath deeply in and out 10 times as slowly as possible.
2) Sit on the floor, with back straight, legs stretched out in front of you, arms straight and the palm of your hands flat on the floor behind your buttocks.
3) Flex your knees slightly, and while you breathe in slowly, lift your pelvis so that the knees are at the same height as the shoulders.
4) Stay in this position for 5 seconds, until you've finished breathing in.
Repeat the exercise 5 times until you can do it 30 times a day. Every two days do it two more times. If after a few buttock-lifts you feel your

head spinning, it is important to rest for a couple minutes: the hyper-oxygenation effect will pass immediately.

Using exercise machines

In addition to the exercises to do at home, there is also some equipment, not bulky and easy to use, which enables you to tone up specific, critical areas more effectively.

INNER THIGH FIRMER
Useful for firming up the inner muscles of the thighs, i.e. the muscles that enable us to keep our knees together. The skin on the inner thighs will appear smoother and firmer.

It is used in an upright position, with your back against a hard surface (back of a chair, chair or wall). With the two outer parts placed between your knees, you try to press your thighs together. The exercise must be repeated at least 5 times a day.

MINISTEPPER
This machine stimulates stairclimbing. It works the muscles of the calves, the extensor and flexor muscles of the legs and the buttocks, making thighs and buttocks firmer.

Part Four

With the doctor's help
Therapies

Anticellulite therapies

Not always are dieting and exercising enough by themselves to solve the problems connected to cellulite in its more advanced stages. This is why the need arises to resort to therapies which can be applied only by a specialist, by means of a visit to a doctor who will help each person choose the therapy best suited to their specific problem.

The most common and effective methods used to eliminated even the toughest kinds of cellulite are *mesotherapy, ultrasound therapy* (often both are combined), *laser therapy, magnetic therapy* and *elect o-toning therapy.*

Mesotherapy

Mesotherapy is a technique which enables small doses of drugs diluted in sterile solutions to be injected hypodermically, so that the solution can penetrate to the area affected by cellulite using a very thin needle, no longer than 1/2 cm. Injecting these substances produces inflammatory mechanisms which help restore the local blood circulation.

Since the underlying cause of all cellulite disorders involves a vascular factor, which causes an alteration in the microcirculation due to a genetic predisposition and many sources of lymphatic stagnation (overly tight clothes, sedentary lifestyle, unbalanced diet, smoking, high heels) generally the first sessions begin with the injection of *phlebotonic,* which have a vasoprotective effect, especially when the person has varicose veins and capillaries in the legs.

In the event that there is a prevalence of adipose tissue, i.e. fat tissue, *xantinic based* drugs are used, which have a lipolytic effect. Generally, women tend to gain weight in the hips and thighs, and it is here that such drugs are utilized; they stimulate the loosening of the fat cells and aid in draining the liquid from the interstitial cells. This is why during the first sessions there may be an increase in diuresis, especially during the half hour following the session.

At times patients are afraid of feeling pain; actually, the treatment does involve some pain, but by using a local anesthetic the discomfort may easily be offset. Mesotherapy can also be applied in cases of accumulated fat in the abdomen, hips, arms, calves and ankles. Its effect is enhanced if followed by ultrasound therapy.

Small *quantities* of medicinal substances are used so as to avoid toxic effects, and this allows the region affected by the disorder to be treated directly.

The needles utilized vary in length from 0.4 mm to 4 mm.

Following the injection, the arterioles of the area treated dilate, which improves circulation and thus facilitates the therapeutic processes.

Ultrasounds

Ultrasounds are waves that vibrate at a frequency above the threshold of human hearing, which is 20,000 Hz. They are used in ultrasound scanning, physiotherapy, to grind up kidney stones, and in esthetic medicine for treating cellulite.

The ultrasounds employed in this therapy have a frequency of 3 MHz, which is 3,000,000 **Hertz** and a variable intensity of 2.0 and 3.0 W sq. cm.

If used with proper equipment and under medical supervision, ultrasounds are not painful. They are transmitted through transducers, round and flat heads (above on right) which are placed on the skin and left there for 15 to 30 minutes according to need.

They are painless and above all are not invasive in that no needles are used. The patient only feels a pleasant sensation of warmth.

There is undoubtedly a compound mechanism. The first macroscopic effect, visible even on the skin surface, is a reactive vasoldilatation, a complicated term to indicate the redness of the skin that can be seen when it is exposed to a source of heat. This effect is useful for increasing the local circulation of blood especially in the areas affected by cellulite, which by antonomasia are characterized by a chronic lack of oxygen due to the scarse blood circulating there (stagnant hypoxia).

The lymphatic vessels, which are like water-scooping pumps with the role of draining the liquids in between the cells, are thus stimulated both indirectly, as a reaction to the dialtion of the blood vessels, and directly, because the ultrasounds cause the lymph nodes to get rid of the liquid they have soaked up. The result is the elimination of both excess liquid and the fibrous tissue deposited in the cellulitic tissue, in addition to a greater oxygen supply to the disabled cells.

Another direct, exquisitely mechanic effect is that produced by the impact of the ultrasounds on the fibrous tissue that acts as the scaffolding of cellulite. Do not panic, there is no quick and dangerous action, but rather a slow and harmless one. The energy transmitted to the cells could cause a reduction in the energy material (glycerol and fatty acids) contained in it in the form of triglycerides.

This fact is substantiated by the evidence that if we apply ultrasounds to a piece of lard, it melts as if it were exposed to heat.

The action of the ultrasounds at this particular frequency is limited to the first 2.5 centimeters of tissue.

In the presence of fat deposits alone, a good diet is enough to eliminate the problem of excess weight once and for all, but along with fat, more often than not, there is fibrous tissue that suffocates the capillaries of the adipose tissue, preventing adequate circulation, causing the area to become painful and ugly bumps to appear on the skin surface which give it that 'orange peel' or 'matress' look typical of cellulite.

The right therapy should be aimed at solving this problem without damaging the healthy tissue and without causing the patient any pain. Ultrasounds enable these objectives to be achieved already during the initial sessions.

The skin will look lighter, less shiny and less puffy. The reddish blotches, a sign of poor circulation, and the heaviness and swelling in the legs will begin to subside rapidly.

The results will be even more amazing if, in the case of obesity, the patient returns to a normal weight, without overly rapid weight loss but with a constant loss of 500 grams every week.

For example, by losing one kilo, an average of one centimeter is lost from the thighs, but if ultrasound therapy is combined with dieting, as many as three can be lost.

In order to implement a proper therapeutic program, it is especially important to estimate the presence or absence of a conspicuous edematous component (filled with water), because in these cases it is essential to include lymphodrainage, still with ultrasounds, but which affects all the lymph stations of the legs and pelvic region; therefore, it is useful to start with a series of sessions (generally 8-10) on a weekly basis, under strict medical supervision and evaluating with the thermographic method the progress of the therapy and areas stil affected by celulite, so as to carry out a targeted therapy.

Obviously, event his technique would not have great results if, in the cases of third and fourth degree cellulite (where there is liquid and fibrous tissue), the therapy were not combined with mesotherapy, with single needle, and the general medical treatment of cellulite.

In my vast case record, I have been able to observe that this technique is successful in all the stages of cellulite and that in the first three stages there is a total remission.

One last application has proven to be the premenstrual syndrome, where there is a certain amount of swelling and tension in the skin. In this case, a single session is enough reduce the above symptoms considerably.

Laser therapy

The application of laser rays on infrared bands causes the capillaries and precapillaries to dilate with increased drainage of the interstitial liquid in the area treated.

Laser therapy supplies electromagnetic energy, which has an effect on cell metabolism. Its different applications depend on the wave length required by the affected tissue. It is, moreover, a biostimulator since it induces cells to react.

The laser used is with infrareds and may be monodiodic or penta-diodoc, controlled by a microprocessor. It serves to increase the flow of blood in the areas affected by cellulite, bringing more oxygen to those specific areas and allowing the lymphatic vessels to reabsorb the liquid from the tissue.

An IR diode laser is also used for lipodystrophy. In the tissue affected by cellulite, especially in the third and fourth stages, the blood flow is reduced, so the area affected receives less oxygen and the irritating fiber accumulates even more. The action carried out by laser therapy on fourth-degree cellulite is seen in its various effects:

1) with an analgesic effect (painless), because it affects the nerve ends blocking the pain stimuli, acting on the sodium-potassium pump of the nerve end, thus allowing an exchange of electrolytes essential for regulating the impulse;

2) with an antiphlogistic effect (which counteracts inflammation);

3) with an antiedema effect, speeding up the blood flow;

4) with a regenerating effect, acting on the cell exchanges and stimulating, whenever necessary, the healing process in damaged tissue.

If used in combination with mesotherapy, laser therapy enhances the pharmacological action, renders the capillaries less fragile and reduces hematic overflow.

It has a disintoxicating effect on irritating metabolites (lactic acid) which cause pain after intense physical exercise. In the fourth stage of celulite these metabolites are drained with greater difficulty. With the laser rays, the circulation becomes more fluid again, the connective tissue is drained more quickly and the edema tends to dissipate gradually and disappear.

The obnoxious pain caused by the interstitial liquid retained in the tissues that make the skin puffy and shiny also disappears.

The laser infrareds work on the affected area by increasing the cell metabolism and the consumption of energy, i.e. acting as a biostimulator. Moreover, it speeds up the microvascular and lymphatic flow in the cellulitic area, acting as a biostimulator of the tissue in which the phlogosis is present.

In my patients, I apply laser therapy after a mesotherapy session, particularly when the person a predisposed to fragile capillaries.

The laser is a highly useful device when the area affected by cellulite is painful, as is always the case in the fourth stage. The patient feels the benefit especially when going to bed at night, sleeping on the part of the body that was treated. After the laser therapy, the area feels less hard, with less water retention and is less painful. The persistent pain that accompanied fourth degree cellulite is relieved and finally disappears already during the first sessions.

Magnetic therapy

This is a technique based on the influence that a magnetic force exerts on an organism; it has been used for many years in osteopathic disorders and is also utilized in traumatology for fractures, in orthopedic medicine for arthrosis and in dermatology for scars.

In the field of cellulite it is used to stimulate circulation, reduce inflammation in affected tissues and increase cellular exchanges. In the event that there is a loss of muscle tone, a considerable difference can be seen, especially in the inner thigh region.

Caption pg. 205

THE MAGNETIC FIELD

Is a force field created by both magnets and electric currents. Our body is also magnetic and feels the action (induction) exerted on it from a distance by bodies with electric or magnetic properties. Magnetic induction is measured in gauss or tesla. (1 tesla=10,000 gauss)

Even on the skin surface, an increase in skin tone will be seen and the skin will appears more elastic. The principle this technique is based on consists in increasing the speed of the blood flow by micromassage and stimulating the exchange of local nutrients. Creating a magnetic field, this therapy is used with caution if the patient has metal protheses and is not employed in women who have inserted a spiral.

It is utilized by athletes for rapid psycho-physical recovery, because it appears to also have an effect on psychological mood and stress.

Electro-toning therapy

Electro-toning therapy is used to counteract a loss of skin tone.

It is a technique that employs electric currents to bring about ionic movements. In this way it causes a superficial vasodilatation and a reddish appearance on the skin, which is a sign of increased blood flow, both in the skin and muscles.

The simulative devices, by means of electric impulses, induce muscle contractions similar to those obtained during physical exercise, reproducing the nervous stimulation of the muscles. Thus the muscles are not simply compressed, but actually contract, which enables the muscles and the skin in that area to become firmer, and restores the tone that was lost in the area treated, in addition to burning up the local fat. There is one kind, that can be bought at a pharmacy, to complete the toning therapy at home (see central photo). The type used by specialists (see photo below) has more sophisticated applications.

Electro-toning therapy is used along with other types of anticellulite therapies whenever the cellulitic and adipose tissue is accompanied by loss of tone in the tissue.

Stretch marks

These are very frequent in women who have lost weight. After losing several kilos, ugly white lines, called stretch marks, may appear on the skin of the abdomen, thighs and arms.

All women fear them, because it is difficult to reduce the number and size of these lines.

Stretch marks are linear depressions that may be either red or white. The width of the marks varies from a few millimeters to 2 centimeters, and may be anywhere from 1 to 20 centimeters long. In the *inflammatory phase,* they take on a reddish hue, while in the final, cicatrizing, stage, they will have a whitish color. If these white marks are longer than 2 mm it is very difficult for them to disappear completely.

Often stretch marks appear without the parson feeling any particular symptoms, but sometimes there is a slight itching or burning sensation.

The *causes* of stretch marks include puberty, pregnancy, Cushing syndrome (increase in hydrocortisones), cortisone treatments, unbalanced diet with large variations in weight.

To prevent them it is important to use creams that contain elastin, placenta and

---

PLACENTA

Placenta is an extremely purified, natural substance of human origin and for this reason has less probability of causing allergies (hypoallergenic). It is used in esthetic medicine to revitalize skin that is wrinkled and lacking tone, and to remove the veil of fatigue that at times suffocates it.

Placenta extract contains the following components. amino acids, mucopolisaccharides, collagen and nucleic acids. These are the basic elements required by the skin to naturally synthesize its own collagen, and they can be compared to the bricks and cement that are added to the supporting framework: our skin. Placenta has the role of nourishing the cells and supplying all the essential elements they require to improve the cell functions and which constitute a real energy supplement_ Placenta is also used in general medicine for its cicatrizing and regenerating effect on tissue damaged by wounds or burns.

Targeted placenta therapy helps moisturize the skin and thus to appear fresher.

collagen, to keep the skin elastic. During pregnancy an anti-stretch mark cream is useful after the third month.

To alleviate and, in certain cases, reduce the number of stretch marks, there are different therapies depending on the seriousness of the problem.

THERAPY FOR RED-PINK STRETCH MARKS. r

1) Placenta injections along the streak, creating microponfett .
2) Then, application of infrared laser therapy to eliminate inflammation and edema.

The tissue treated in this manner will begin to synthesize its own collagen.

THERAPY FOR WHITE STRETCH MARKS

1) Applications of 70% glycolic acid along the marks for 2-5 minutes according to each person's sensitivity.
2) After this, counteract the effect of the acid with a neutralizing solution.
3) Hypodermic collagen injections with a product containing placenta. Locally, the inflammatory reaction will cause the blood to circulate better and stimulate the production of collagen, so as to fill the hollow streak. The color also tends to become more uniform with the surrounding skin.

For perfect breasts

One of my patients asked me: 'Why is it that in the past when I lost even a little weight my breasts got smaller, but now I don't see such a big difference?'.

To answer this question, I have to provide some background information on the anatomic and functional configuration of breasts and on the kinds of treatment that help improve their appearance.

The breasts are located on the *greater pectoral* muscle and are situated between the muscle and the skin. It is composed of a *mammary gland*, formed of 15-20 wedge-shaped lobes with ducts at their ends called *galactophorous ducts*, which have the function of bringing the secretion of the gland to the nipple. Between the lobes there is connective tissue which supports the entire gland.

The rest of the breast is composed of adipose tissue, which fills and protects the gland from external trauma.

The *consistency* and the *hardness* of the breasts, therefore, depends on the elasticity of the connective tissue and by the amount of fatty tissue.

During the *menstrual cycle*, after ovulation (after the 14th day), the mammary is enlarged by 15-45 cubic centimeters due to the female sex hormones, estrogen and progesterone. This increase in volume is caused by the proliferation of the galactophorous ducts. The breasts reach their maximum degree of enlargement during the premenstrual period and then become smaller around the seventh day of the cycle.

During *pregnancy*, the increase of the galactophorous ducts, especially in the last months, is permanent. Unlike before, however, there is a reduction in the amount of connective tissue, so the breasts appear flabbier, as the fat component is more prevalent (this change is necessary, because the function of the breasts during pregnancy is to prepare for breastfeeding, and excessive connective tissue would cause pain).

The *turgidity* of the breasts, therefore, is determined by their glandular component, and this explains why it may vary during the life cycle of a woman (menstrual cycle, pregnancy, breastfeeding, menopause).

It is clear that there is no is no other method apart from administering hormones orally or locally that can increase the galactophoroous ducts of the mammary glands, and therefore, since *hormone* treatments are very delicate, they should be prescribed by an endocrinologist for particular cases.

The only components that can be improved upon without causing any damage, and providing good results, are the *connective tissue*, the muscle *component* and the *fatty* tissue.

Regarding the *connective* tissue *component*, there are a number of skin treatments, using creams and lotions, that we can classify according to their function:

1) products *containing substances* that halt the degeneration *of collagen and* elastin, the chief constituents of connective tissue: plant proteinic extract having a high anti-collagenase enzyme action, organic silicon compounds, glycose amino glycans, vitamin E and retinene;

2) products that act selectively on the fibrillary *and* elastic structures *of* the epidermis: extracts of alchemilla, salvia,equisetum,hedera agrimoniu, bearberry, algae, ginseng, ginkgo biloba, plant DNA;

3) precursors *of* collagen: extracts of human placenta. This contains amino acids, mucopolysaccharides, collagen and nucleic acids.

Regarding the muscle *component*, secondly, it has been found that physical exercise is the best treatment. As already mentioned, the breasts rest on the greater pectoral muscle. This muscle should be worked for at least half an hour a day, by doing some simple exercises during breaks at work or finding the time to do specific exercises. Below are some examples:

1) in the morning, as soon as you wake up, use a cold, moist sponge to tone up the skin, then clamp your hands together 100 times at the height of your breasts and push your hands together. Your breasts will rise;

2) Hold a tennis ball in both hands, lift your elbows to shoulder height and try to

Caption pg. 210

Creams or lotions for the connective tissue Exercises for the pectoral muscles

squeeze the ball with your hands. Repeat the exercise 20 times a day;

3) standing in front of a wall, rest your hands on the wall and bend your arms. Repeat 30 times a day.

Regarding the *fat component,* it is important to remember that a crash diet may have a negative influence on the bosom. The breasts, in fact, are composed chiefly of adipose tissue. Given this fact, it is obvious that an uncontrolled loss or increase in weight may damage the shapeliness of the breasts, whose form and firmness depend on the quantity of fat present.

Variations in weight of more than 4 kilos over a brief period may reduce the volume of the breasts and make them less firm. Women who are obese are even more at risk. They will have to be very careful not to lose more than 4-5 kilos per month; only in this way does the skin have enough time to adapt and the breasts will not sag.

A specialist will determine the degree and especially the type of obesity characterizes the patient (android or gynoid). The problem resides in the fact that, when dieting, women with android obesity loses weight in her breasts and abdomen too, while women with gynoid obesity have difficulty losing weight in their thighs and will lose weight more easily in their breasts and abdomen. Therefore, in both cases, the solution lies in following a diet that is not too drastic.

In general, the women who are most preoccupied with their breasts are those with obesity in the upper part of their body (tummy and bosom), and will often desire plastic surgery to reduce their breast size, not realizing that a general weight loss will also reduce that area by several sizes.

If, instead, the breasts are small, it will be necessary to determine whether the body shape is an android or gynoid type. Of course, if a woman is at her ideal weight or underweight, it will be more difficult to identify what type she is. She can gain 2 or 3 kilos so as to increase the fatty tissue in the breasts, but it is

Caption pg. 21

gash dieting aril for the breasts

advisable to do much exercising to develop the pectoral muscle as well; as this muscle develops and becomes firmer, it will cause the breasts to rise and protrude further.

Many women complain that their breasts are too small, others too big, and often they think they can only solve their problem surgically, without considering that with an appropriate diet they can also obtain substantial improvements.

Considering that a diet for the breasts must necessarily fall within the framework of a general, and highly personalized, diet, it is possible to trace some guidelines applicable to all women:

1) maintain a stable body weight at normal levels;

2) eat a daily amount of noble protein (found in eggs, meat, milk and dairy products, and fish) not less than one gram per kilo of body weight,

3) take vitamins with antioxidant properties (A, C, E), that have the function of preventing the formation of free radicals, which, by now well known, cause an early aging of the skin. For this reason it is recommended to take daily:

—1 tablespoon of wheat germ oil (vitamin E)—1 glass of fresh carrot juice (vitamin A)

—2 kiwis (vitamin C);

4) take the trace element selenium, which has an anti-aging function (the right amount is found in a cup of non-detheinated tea).

The types of diets must be subdivided into three groups: 1) high-calorie diet (weight gain)

2) normal calorie diet (weight maintenance) 3) low-calorie diet (weight loss).

As already mentioned, the breasts are composed mainly of fat. This is the reason why a specialist in nutritional science can help in maintaining or improving their appearance.

When following an unbalanced low-calorie diet, without medical supervision, to

Caption pg. 212

Little hints to enhance the beauty of the breasts

TEA, A PRECIOUS DRINK
The theine contained in in tea is lipolytic, which means it helps dissolve fat.

obtain fast results (for example, 10 kilos in one month), this is where the real problems crop up. If the weight loss is rapid, rarely will the tissues in the body not be affected. Several kilos can be lost, as long as the weight loss does not exceed one kilo per week. Naturally, this limit depends on the predisposition in each individual for tissue recovery. The specialist will also evaluate the elasticity of the skin, so as to prevent the breasts from sagging, with an internal treatment that predominantly involves a diet, and external treatment involving electro-toning therapy, exercises or cosmetic products such as creams and lotions.

The fat in the breasts can be lost only by reducing the amount of Calories, whereas the muscles can be modified with a correct diet that combines protein and carbohydrates, because protein, in order to be used in building up the muscles, needs the right amount of carbohydrates. Eating only protein does not build up the connective tissue since it is then used as energy instead of the missing glucides. In order to increase the volume of the pectoral muscle, therefore, the protein that is eaten will cement better if combined with the carbohydrates found in bread and pasta.

Below are two examples of menus containing balanced amounts of protein, carbohydrates and vitamins, and which can be used when, in addition to losing weight, a woman also wants to do something for her breasts:

Menu

BREAKFAST *Milk or coffee*

SNACK KIWI
LUNCH *Rice 70 gr+1 spoonful of Parmesan* To PREPARE *Boil the rice in a saucepan with the peas. When done, sprinkle with Parmesan. Frozen or canned peas 50 gr Radicchio+1 teaspoon of oil*

SNACK A cup of tea
DINNER *Barley soup*
Pearled barley 50 gr • Half a carrot • Half a leek, diced TO PREPARE *Chop the vegetables, add in water and barley and cook slowly until the barley is done.*
Low-fat cheese 150 gr Plenty of lettuce+1 spoon of olive oil vinegar and lemon juice.

Appendix

Caption pg. 71

POTASSIUM CONTENT IN SOME FOODS
(mg of potassium per 100 gr., with non-edible parts removed)

white bread	*125*
whole grain bread	*250-350*
pasta	*160*
rice	*100*
dried beans	*1200*
chickpeas	
fresh broad beans	*325*
dried broad beans	*700*
lentils	*700-1200*
fresh peas	*400*
dried peas	*1000*
asparagus	*200*
artichokes	*430*
carrots	*300*
cabbage and broccoli	*400*
Brussels sprouts	*450*
savoy	*290*
chicory	*400*
onions	*200*
fennel	*410*
endive	*350*
lettuce	*200*
egg plant	*240*
potatoes	*400-600*
ripe tomatoes	*300*
parsley	*700*
celery	*280*
spinach	*500*
apricots	*450*

pineapple	225
oranges	180
bananas	400
cherries	260
figs	225
pears	145
peaches	200
plums	170
grapes	250
milk	150-175
fat and lean meats	350
giblets	300
fish	200-350
cheese	100-150
eggs	150
dark chocolate	450
milk chocolate	400
cocoa	900

Caption pg. 73

A DIURETIC VEGETABLE BROTH

It is easy to prepare. Ingredients: two artichokes, one carrot, one potato.
Boil in two liters of water for half an hour and strain.
ARTICHOKES stimulate the **production of bile (choleretic effect), helps** *the*
evacuation of the intestine(cholagogue effect) and aids diuresis.
CARROTS are rich in vitamin A, which, even after being cooked, is not altered sub-
stantially. They are useful in cases of enteritis (intestinal inflammation).
POTATOES are rich in potassium and stimulate dieresis.

LYMPHODRAINAGE

This technique enables liquids to be drained from the tissue through the lymphatic vessels.
Ultrasound theraav pg. 201-03 Mesotherany
pg. 200-01

Caption pg. 81

MAGNESIUM CONTENT OF SOME FOODS
(mg of magnesium per 100 gr, with non-edible parts removed)
milk

many vegetables fish in general ham and salame meat in general
from 13 to 50 mg
many kinds of cheese polished rice
white bread
from 51 to 80 mg spinach parmesan cheese whole wheat bread
lentils dried figs
from 81 to 100 mg

	over 100 mg
dried beans	*130-180*
dried peas	*120*
soya	*235*
whole grain rice	*120*

For her high triglyceride level, polyunsaturated fatty acids.

For her poor digestion, papaw.

To reduce the amount of fat absorption in the intestines, I gave her *chitosan,* useful both in cases of hypertriglyceridemia and for diets in which less fat must be absorbed.

For her high cholesterol, garcinia cambogia was particularly effective.

To increase diuresis and for an antioxidant effect, *green* tea.

External therapy

Concerning the therapy for her legs, I advised my patient to wait until she had reached her weight loss goal, because I was afraid that if I did therapy on her legs right away, they would become too thin compared to the rest of her body.

Her thighs were well proportioned, so I waited to see the difference in them once she had lost 22 kilos before deciding on the most suitable therapy. They had, in fact, a considerable adipose content, so her weight loss had the result of reducing the diameter of her thighs by about ten centimeters. The cellulite had become evident with deep bulges, because the fat that was holding it in had dissolved, enabling me to diagnose fourth degree cellulite.

It is always preferable to utilize localized therapy in the beginning when treating for people with a gynecoid type distribution of fat and cellulite. Otherwise, as was the case with Marinella, if the therapy is applied before a considerable amount of weight has been lost from dieting, there is a risk that the circumference of the thighs could be reduced too much, since the therapy accelerates the fat dissolving process.

The therapies I used for Marinella included *ultrasounds* on the sides of her

Caption pg. 142

<u>*Ultrasounds*</u> pg. *201-03* <u>*Mesotherapv*</u> pg. *200-01*

0-595-24564-1